The African American Woman's

GUIDE TO

Successful Makeup and Skincare

Revised Edition

Alfred Fornay

AN AMBER BOOK

John Wiley & Sons, Inc.

Copyright © 2002 by Alfred Fornay. All rights reserved
Foreword copyright © 2002 by John Ledes

Published by John Wiley & Sons, Inc., New York
Published simultaneously in Canada

Design and production by Navta Associates, Inc.

Produced by Amber Books, Tony Rose, Publisher, Editorial Director; Samuel P. Peabody, Associate Publisher; Yvonne Rose, Senior Editor

The dosages from the table on page 20 are extrapolated from data in *Life Extension, a Practical Scientific Approach: Adding Years to Your Life and Life to Your Years* by Durk Pearson and Sandy Shaw, copyright © 1982. Reprinted by permission of Warner Books, New York.

ISBN: 0-471-40278-8

Printed in the United States of America
10 9 8 7 6 5 4 3 2

Contents

See the Fornay Color Chart in the middle of the book

Foreword

Al Fornay's first work on beauty and grooming appeared in the *New York Times Magazine*, under the supervision of Patrica Petersen, then fashion editor. The article marked the first recognition of the huge African American color cosmetics market.

Mr. Fornay emerged as one of the recognized authorities on fashion, beauty, and grooming. A graduate of the State University of New York's Fashion Institute of Technology and the City College of New York, with degrees in merchandising and marketing, Mr. Fornay has influenced the marketing and sales strategies of major cosmetics firms such as Fashion Fair, Clairol, and Revlon. His training seminars for sales personnel and beauty consultants helped establish these companies as leaders in beauty and grooming for the African American woman.

While traveling and presenting his seminars throughout the United States, as well as in Canada, London, Paris, and the Caribbean, Fornay developed the unique ability to anticipate the fashion and beauty needs of African American women and men. He was among the first to perceive their desire for quality. Al Fornay helped his readers and advisees to feel and look better.

Fornay's coupling of language with graphic visual images soon had publishing houses seeking his flair for design and service marketing. Mr. Fornay helped the Johnson Publishing Company to establish their Fashion Fair Cosmetics line in Marshall Field's, Bloomingdale's, Carsons, Rich's, Robinsons, J.L. Hudson, Jordan Marsh, Nieman Marcus, Nordstrom, Macy's, and others. Mr. Fornay served as beauty editor at *Ebony* magazine, the first such post conceived to train black women and men in fashion and grooming techniques.

Fornay helped Johnson Publishing Company launch *EM: Ebony Man* magazine, and served as its editor in chief. He also served as the first male beauty editor of *Essence* magazine. And at McGraw-Hill, for *Business Week Careers* magazine, he was a contributing writer in fashion and beauty, an indication to young career seekers that dressing for success is a must.

This book marks Mr. Fornay's leadership as the fashion authority for all African American women.

John Ledes, publisher,
Beauty Fashion magazine and *Cosmetic World* newsletter

Preface

This revised edition of my beauty book was designed, photographed, and written especially for you—women whose skin color ranges from the fair to the darker end of the spectrum. Having read hundreds of beauty books, I realize that much of the information relating to those skin colors is confusing and often dead wrong. So, after more than twenty-five years in the beauty business, I wanted to make sure that all advice and how-to instructions were up-to-date.

Our fabulous cover has already gotten rave reviews from the publisher, booksellers, and beauty, image, and grooming authorities across the country. My unique color chart is still the only one of its kind . . . and I know—from the many letters and cards you have written to me sharing your new beauty experiences—that it is working for you.

Although I focus on African American women, there are millions of other women whose coloring falls into that range: African, Caribbean, Asian, Hispanic, and so on. If you are one of those women, this book is for you. It is about the health and beauty of your skin, its maintenance, its treatment, and its makeup. It is about the application of color to your skin and your nails. This is a "how-to" book for the person of color, whether she's a manager of a small store or an executive of a multimillion-dollar corporation. It is for the secretary of a five-person office and the editor of a major magazine. And perhaps most of all, it is for the homemaker whose jobs are many and whose hours are ongoing. The book is for all women of color who want to look great and take better care of their skin.

Makeup and adornment, particularly the use of color, has a unique significance for black women. The use of makeup is a socioreligious, socioeconomic, and sociopsychological choice as much as it is a beauty choice. You will find some black women going to a cosmetics counter, looking at a photograph of Tyra Banks, Jada Pinkett Smith, Iman, Toni Braxton, Halle Berry, Diahann Carroll, Angela Bassett, Vanessa L. Williams and Whitney Houston and saying, "Oh, I would love to look like that."

A beauty adviser or cosmetologist then attempts to make the woman up "to look like that," and the woman looks at herself in the mirror and says, "Oh no! That's not me." More than likely, the cosmetologist is stunned by this reaction and wonders, what does the woman really want?

Celebrity photographs do not reflect the reality of the woman at the counter. If she is a churchgoing woman, she probably only wears some foundation, shaded powder, tint-type lipstick, and little else. But if she is a top executive in the record industry, then she might be fully made up with color.

A woman's use of color relates to her sense of self and how she interacts with the world. Many African American men don't like their wives or partners using much makeup and color, and this, too, has an effect on how these women appear. In fact, more than 65 percent of the 18 million African American women in the United States have never put color on their faces. (A surprising statistic that should have cosmetic companies wetting their lips!) The question is, though, why don't they wear color and how can they be persuaded to? The makeup section of this book addresses this question and gives the black woman makeup color options that will comfortably suit her sense of self, style, and needs for home, church, social events, and work.

Many cosmetics companies have done outstanding research on how makeup relates to black skin. I will introduce you to their products and research. In this book you will learn how to evaluate the quality of their lines and the many other beauty products filling the shelves of department stores, chain stores, and pharmacies. You will discover how to choose what works best for you. You will learn how to address your own needs, not those of the sales personnel, and be secure in your selection of color for your skin and nails. You will be able to determine your skin type and what colors are appropriate for each season. You will know what corrective beauty products to buy and what regular skincare regimen to follow. And the all-new before and after transformations are for your future beauty knowledge and review. By the time you finish reading this book, you will know the state of the art in the beauty industry and how to use that knowledge to your advantage.

I believe that every black woman is beautiful. She just needs to know how to present her beauty. After reading this book, you will be able to do just that. You will be confident, knowledgeable, well-groomed, fabulous, and successful!

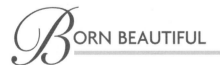 ORN BEAUTIFUL

African American women are beautiful. All women of color are born beautiful, but a larger percentage have made themselves even more beautiful thanks to the skilled use of cosmetics. For the past several years, many professional cosmetic educators have criss-crossed our nation teaching and instructing women of color in the proper application of cosmetics to their faces: Byron Barnes, Roxanna Floyd, Ellie Winslow, Reggie Wells, Sheila Evers, James Harris, Katara, Ricci, Bert Emmanuel, Lumus Hamilton, Lazarus, Ashley Hall, Kirk Norris Harris, D'angelo Thompson, Jonathan Romania, and, most recently, Sam Fine and Christopher Michael.

We have all taught young and mature women that when properly applied, makeup can bring radiance to your complexion and smooth, conceal, or camouflage your flaws. It can even change the shape of your face. All of the professional beauty educators advise this, but makeup must be used with wisdom and discretion. That little touch of color here and pat of powder there can read like a billboard, telling the world about a woman's fashion savvy, her personal grooming habits, and her good taste.

The strong and beautiful "women with substance," featured on the following pages, are representative of successful African American women. Susan Taylor, Sylvia Rhone, Terrie Williams, and Kelly Price are four out of the billions of women who are born beautiful, including you. These women, along with the other featured personalities who come from all walks of life, whose bios and beauty regimens grace the opening page of each chapter, were selected for this book because they exemplify women of color from all over the world. Their natural beauty combined with intelligence, education, spirituality, and a professional image makes these women champions in every way.

This book will help you to enhance your natural beauty by achieving and maintaining flawless skin through the dedicated use of skincare products and the appropriate application of makeup. I wish you well. Remain beautiful and strong, always.

Yours in spirit,
Alfred Fornay

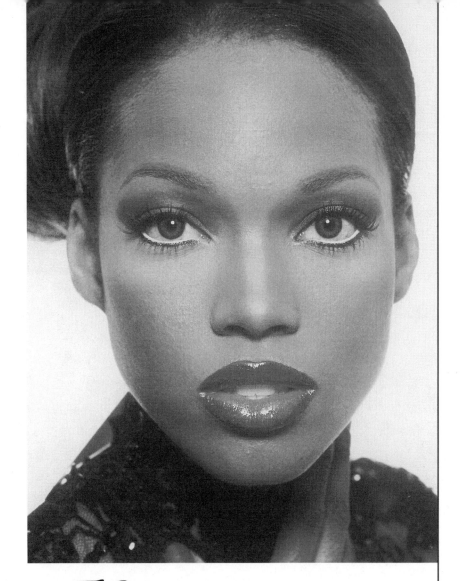

HOW YOUR SKIN PROTECTS YOU

1

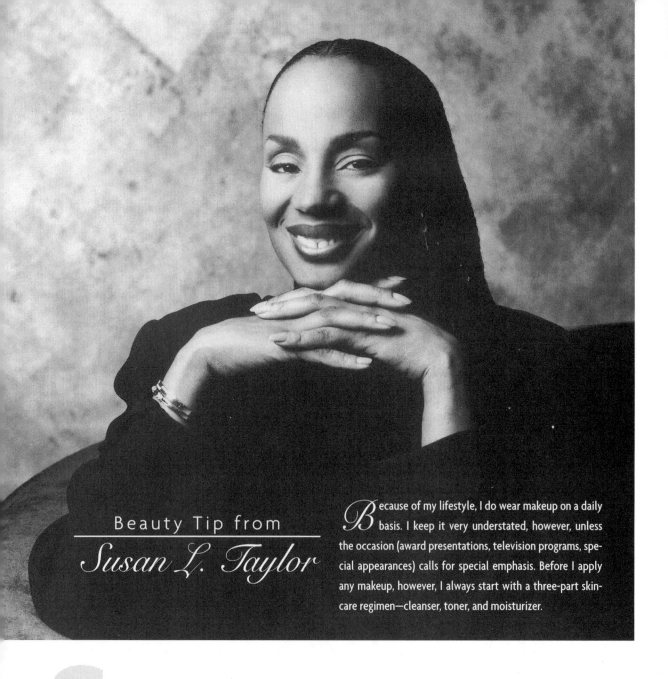

Beauty Tip from
Susan L. Taylor

*B*ecause of my lifestyle, I do wear makeup on a daily basis. I keep it very understated, however, unless the occasion (award presentations, television programs, special appearances) calls for special emphasis. Before I apply any makeup, however, I always start with a three-part skin-care regimen—cleanser, toner, and moisturizer.

Susan L. Taylor is publication director for *Essence* magazine. As former editor in chief, she guided *Essence* through a period of phenomenal growth. Her acclaimed monthly editorials, "In the Spirit," led Susan to the publication of a series of books—*In the Spirit: The Inspirational Writings of Susan L. Taylor, Lessons in Living,* and *Confirmation and the Spiritual Wisdom That Has Shaped Our Lives* (coauthored by her husband, Khephra Burns).

Your skin can be your best friend. It is your confidante. It is your protector. It takes all types of abuse, and yet it is quickly ready to forgive.

Your skin is a multifaceted creation that can't be duplicated by human beings. It keeps out the harsh external environment—that is, germs and bacteria—while it protects your vital organs. It helps maintain your body temperature by preventing heat from escaping too rapidly, which would be harmful or even fatal. Your skin stores nutrients for future protection.

Your skin is versatile and sensitive. It reacts to stress, pain, illness, pleasure, and happiness as well as to light and dark, hot and cold. It stretches and shrinks, wrinkles and unwrinkles. It needs minimal but regular, consistent, and thorough attention if you want it to show you at your very best. But for all your skin's strength and versatility, today it is under siege. It was not constructed to withstand being bombarded by today's natural and unnatural stresses.

GEOGRAPHY AND THE SEASONS

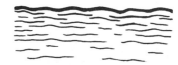

Where you live has a direct effect on your skin, particularly on your face, which is almost always exposed to the elements. Your face has an upper, or outer, layer of skin called the epidermis. This layer is what you touch and see when you look in the mirror. Another name for this layer, owing to the shape of the cells making up the layers, is the "horny" layer (stratum corneum).

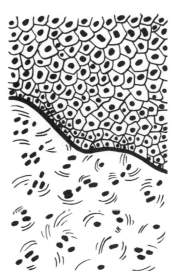

The upper layer of epithelial tissue, the under layer of germinating tissue, and the dermis, with regular blood cells.

Although everyone has this outer skin layer, the thickness of the covering differs from person to person. African Americans have more layers to their epidermis than do whites. But even among blacks, the number of layers varies. Now you can understand why your face, to some degree, reacts differently to the forces assaulting it than do the faces of other women you know. The outermost portion of the epidermis consists of dead cells. That is why sometimes, after washing your face and drying it with a face towel, you may notice flaking skin on your forehead. Your face casts off this outermost layer of skin in pieces. As the outer layer is dispelled, an under-layer takes its place. This process constantly renews your skin. Each outermost layer falls away when it has absorbed all the stress it can manage, and then the underlayer takes its place.

When this surface action is taking place, the underlayer is protected, waiting to supply your face with a new fighting army of cells. Beneath the epidermis is the germinating layer, but before discussing this lower layer, let's see what geography and climate can do to the outer layer of your skin.

If you live in a region that is warm year-round, like California, then your skin will be affected differently than if you live on the East Coast, in a climate that has four varying seasons. Obviously, where your home is determines the amount of the sun and its damaging ultraviolet rays that you will be exposed to. But this is only the beginning.

Office buildings are air-conditioned year-round. When you fly, you are in a pressurized aircraft. The same air is continuously recirculated, sometimes

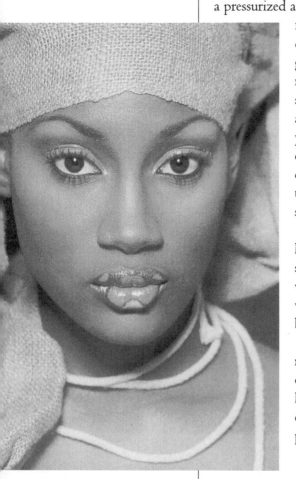

for several hours. Moisture in the air gets lost. The drier air can lead to drier skin. Whether you're in the sky or on the ground, air-conditioning draws humidity from the air and moisture from the skin. Central heating also dries out the skin. These modern conveniences are stressful to your face and trigger the aging process prematurely. If you go from your climate-controlled home or office into a sun-drenched day, you bombard your skin with ultraviolet rays and further draw off moisture. Whenever that happens, your skin really takes a beating. The skin is left dry, peeling, and if the exposure was too intense, with its underlayers damaged.

This is the damage that sunburns do: you peel or you're left with leathery-looking skin. Worse, this constant negative stress breaks down the face's connective tissue, resulting in wrinkles and "premature aging." With steady damage, those wrinkles and lines around the eyes and mouth get deeper and become more prominent.

If you live in a seasonally cool or temperate climate, you might feel safer. But wherever you live or work, your skin is often exposed to automobile emissions, major industrial pollutants, and wind. Wind alone can strike at your skin and cause damage, but when that wind carries pollutants, the problem is intensified. The pollutants that cause acid rain destroy forests and crops, so you can imagine the struggle your outer-skin layer has in protecting your body from environmental assaults.

Other natural assaults, such as those from germs, bacteria, and environmental impurities, must also be prevented from getting below the skin's surface. So no matter where you live, your face contends with major stresses. More often than not, the outer layer stands up to these assaults—but at a cost: dryness, wrinkles and lines, and skin disorders. Your skin can't fight the "good fight" alone; it needs your help. *There is hope.*

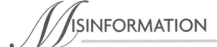ISINFORMATION

Perhaps even more disturbing than the elements our skin is exposed to is the degree to which people are misinformed. Because of their African heritage, black and dark-skinned women and men have often been led to believe that their skin is built for the sun. Though this may seem true, it is in fact not true.

Most "blacks" living in the desert, or in comparably dry, hot regions like the Sudan, almost always totally cover their bodies, leaving very little of their skin exposed to the sun. In contrast, people living in hot, humid areas are apt to wear less clothing—and rightfully so. Generally, the hot, humid areas are less industrialized and have fewer if any direct pollutants, and the humidity in the air reduces the degree to which skin moisture evaporates. People who live in very humid climates don't peel and their skin, whether black or white, often has fewer wrinkles. Their faces belie their age. The outer layer of their skin is moist and pliable, rather than dry and lined.

I've talked with women from Gabon and the Central African Republic, and they complain about how dry their skin becomes when they visit America. Their complaints have validity, since the humidity here is comparatively low. A change in climate like this can often start to affect your skin within a few days or less. So remember—whatever your color, protect your skin or you will pay for the neglect.

Black skin has special qualities. As I noted earlier, it has more epidermal layers than white skin. To some degree, this means greater protection from the sun, and those additional layers often help black skin to appear and feel smoother. Black skin has more melanin (the dark pigment in the epidermis), which reflects more of the sun's rays, giving greater protection and reducing the drying process. But for all these positive qualities, black skin needs as much care as any other if it is to maintain its health and good looks.

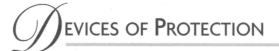

DEVICES OF PROTECTION

Remember, there are two upper layers to the skin: the epidermis and the germination layer, which together make up the skin's essential defense system. The outer layer has two essential ingredients helping it to do its job and maintain its "looks": water and sebaceous oils. These two elements—no matter how often you may have heard that oil and water don't mix—work together beautifully to support and protect the skin.

The epidermis needs water to keep it pliable, plump, and elastic. The body supplies that water through the cells. Later I will discuss diet, but for now I mention only that you need to drink plenty of water to maintain healthy skin. The sebaceous glands produce oils that travel upward and cover the surface of the skin. The oils act as a defensive shield and a reflector, not only holding the skin's surface moisture in but also keeping the skin soft, pliable, and unbroken. However, once moisture is drawn from the outer layer, the oils cannot help restore the skin's youthful quality. Only water will do the job. If you soak a piece of dry skin in oil, for example, it will not soften. It will not soften even if you use sebaceous oil. The oil is not the softener; water is. Remember this principle when we focus on products for your skincare regimen.

Epithelial tissue, the dermis, and a pore opening with a sebaceous gland extending upward to the skin's surface.

THE GERMINATING LAYER

Beneath the epidermis is the germinating layer. Actually, this is the deepest layer of the epidermis, resting on the corium, which is also called the derma, or true skin. But the germinating layer is so different from the rest of the epidermis, and should be nurtured so differently, that I present it as though it were a distinct layer. It consists of a single row of columnar cells in which young cells develop and move upward to the surface.

The top cells making up the germinating layer move upward while others remain, protecting the corium beneath. The germinating layer does not use water or oils to maintain itself but is nourished, by the blood circulated to the skin. This layer of cells is nourished as are cells in the rest of your body, through proper nutrients. This is why what you eat and don't eat, what you take into your system and what you don't take into it, will show in your face. What gets into your circulatory system will be seen, one way or another. Drinking alcohol will show, smoking will show, drugs will show, birth control pills will show. A healthful or poor diet will show. Your skin is an indicator of your state of health. Moreover, your state of health will either help or prevent your skin from doing its job.

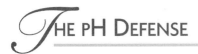HE pH DEFENSE

Those sebaceous glands have another defensive purpose besides holding in the skin's moisture. They maintain what is called an acid mantle across the skin's surface. Healthy skin is slightly acidic. It is believed that skin with a tendency toward alkalinity (the opposite of acidity) is more likely to become infected and have skin disorders. The pH factor of healthy skin (a tendency toward acidity) works as a defense by affecting the skin's ability to both ward off infection and disorders and thereby save the body from having to fight beneath the surface as well. So when you see products proclaiming to return the skin's pH factor, don't automatically accept or reject them, but know that the pH measure is important.

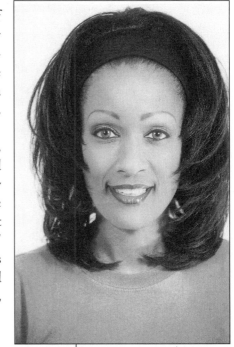

I have deliberately not discussed the skin's corium, or derma, since commercial products cannot affect it. Your genes, diet, and cosmetic surgery are its primary influences. So you can readily understand that the epidermis and germination layers, with the sebaceous glands, are the skin's primary, effective defense against the environment—both man-made and natural. The "falloff" defensive process of the outermost layer of the epidermis serves two vital functions: (1) the older and drier cells are removed, and as the layer of the cells falls off, (2) the environmental impurities, bacteria, and pollutants on or in them are removed.

This self-renewing process is ongoing, with little visible evidence when your skin is young and healthy. However, when your skin is neither young nor healthy, then the process works less effectively, with the noticeable results of lines, wrinkles, cracks, and peeling. But with help and knowledge, you can retard the aging process and keep your skin healthy and youthful-looking.

WATER—A KEY TO YOUTHFUL-LOOKING SKIN

Even though the outer layer of the skin receives a continuous supply of water from the inner layer, the amount provided is limited at any given time. Thus, the outer layer is often short of water when it may need it most. For example, if the skin's loss of water to the atmosphere exceeds its upward supply, then the skin is in danger of going dry. If you don't use a sunscreen or moisturizing guard, the extreme dry conditions in such areas as Arizona, New Mexico, and the desert in California can have a dangerous effect on your skin.

THE AGING PROCESS

If you look at the skin of an older person, particularly if it has been neglected or abused, you will find evidence of structural change. The dead, outer layer of the epidermis is thicker and therefore drier. This is partly because the epidermis of an older person begins to produce a slightly different type of cell.

Furthermore, with age these cells stick together with greater adhesion and are not shed as readily. The outer layers of dead skin begin to build up, becoming thicker and thicker atop the lower, living layers. These outer layers have not only less water or moisture in them but also less capacity to hold water. Unless their moisture capacity is increased, the outer, now thicker layer becomes dry and wrinkled. This causes crepey lines to appear, with the ends of the cells curling up, leading to roughness.

During this aging process, the oil glands decrease in function, with the decline greater in women than in men. Also, the surface guard of oil, whose function is to hold moisture in the skin, does not work as well. Without its water retention, the skin loses its pliability and softness.

SUNTANNING AND THE AGING PROCESS

Tanning is a defense the skin uses to protect its delicate inner layers. The increase in pigment, brought about through exposure to sunlight, is by and large temporary; the suntan disappears in time. However, during the aging process, there is a tendency for these pigments to increase, causing the skin to become darker and, in some instances, blotchy. These darker areas usually appear on the hands and face. Often they are called age spots or liver spots. With continued use, fade cream, gel, and lotion formulas can be an effective method to temporarily fade age spots. But spots will reappear without regular applications. Actually, these are the result of suntanning combined with the aging process. People who stay out of the sun have fewer, if any, liver spots.

LINES, WRINKLES, AND SPOTS

If you were able to take a look at the skin's lower layer—the dermis—you would notice elastic fibers. Unlike the epidermis, or outer layer, the dermis cannot regenerate itself. Any damage done to the dermis results in degeneration and the formation of scar tissue. This means there is a structural change, no matter how slight. It is this underlayer that is responsible for the resiliency of your facial skin, whether smooth and unlined or rough and wrinkled. The dermis is composed of layers of living tissue, and this tissue is permeated with elastic fibers—reinforcement rods that help keep the skin taut. If damage is done to these rods, sagging and wrinkles are often a result.

With the aging process, the underlayer has a tendency to degenerate, often causing these fibers to break into many pieces. Their supportive effec-

PROTECT THOSE LAYERS AND LOOK YOUTHFUL

Remember: when damage occurs in the dermis, in the facial area, or elsewhere, the effects are permanent. Only cosmetic surgery can rebuild or stretch the perception of new life and youth. No matter how much care is given to the face, some structural changes will occur. But these changes can be kept to a minimum with proper care and preventive treatment. This means that paying attention to both the outer and inner layers of the skin is essential.

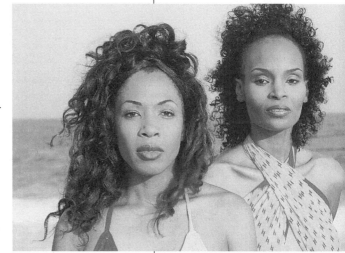

tiveness is then gone, and the dermis is then incapable of "standing up" by itself. In some places, the structure caves in, and the outer surface falls into the crevices. These are the face's grooves, lines, and wrinkles. The skin around the eyes and on the neck is the most likely to show these aging signs first, with the rest of the face showing the effects later.

The blood vessels, which are also in the dermis, expand with age, and little capillaries may even break, causing discoloration.

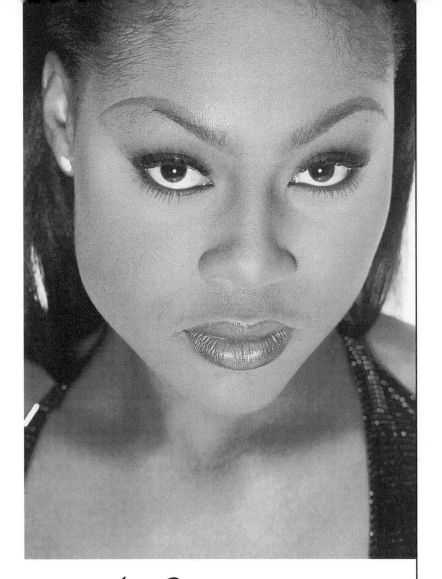

NUTRITION AND YOUR SKIN

2

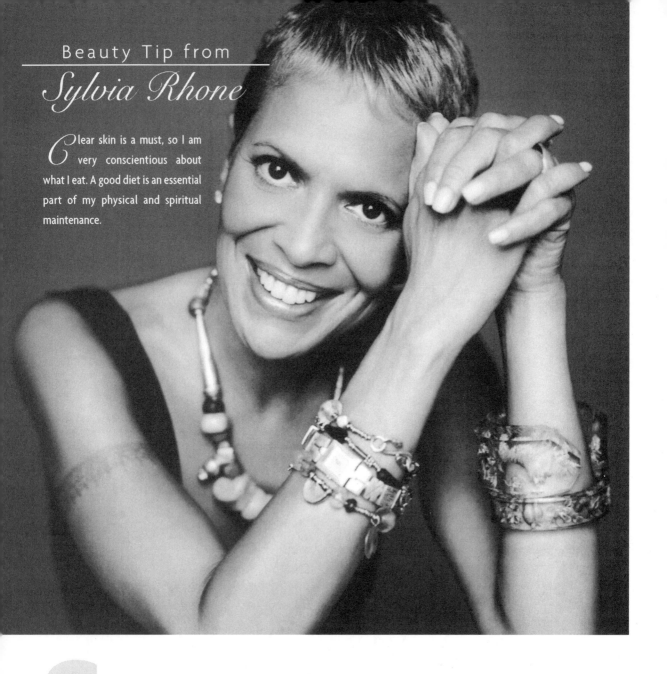

Beauty Tip from
Sylvia Rhone

*C*lear skin is a must, so I am very conscientious about what I eat. A good diet is an essential part of my physical and spiritual maintenance.

Sylvia Rhone's current tenure as chairman of the Elektra Entertainment Group is her latest achievement in a distinguished more than twenty-year career in the music business. Her historic appointment as chairman/CEO of EEG establishes her as the only African American and the first woman in the history of the recording industry to attain such a title.

Let's look at the things you can do to achieve healthier, more youthful skin. A low-fat, high carbohydrate diet is best. Carbohydrates are low in calories and provide energy with other vitamins and minerals. When too much fat is consumed, it usually turns into body fat, and is stored in all the wrong places, including the hips and stomach. Eat foods high in fiber, such as whole grain cereals and bread, pasta, vegetables, beans, nuts, and fruits. Combine herb teas and fruit juices for some good essential vitamins and drink lots of water. And, avoid foods that are too high in saturated fat, cholesterol, sodium, and sugar.

Changing your eating habits takes a lot of discipline, but if you motivate yourself, it's easy to develop a new attitude toward food. Good health, glorious hair, and a glowing complexion are the rewards of a carefully planned diet. Let's review some of the vitamin resources for the foods that you eat.

*F*OOD: THE SOURCE OF NATURAL VITAMINS AND MINERALS

To ensure a balanced diet, meal plans for adults should involve eating a variety of foods from the following groups: vegetables, fruits, whole grains and grain products, yogurt, cheese and milk products; fish, poultry, and meats; beans and peas and other legumes. Having a balanced diet will go a long way toward providing the vitamins and minerals for your overall good health. We have recommended some popular sources.

GOOD SOURCES OF NUTRIENTS

- Pantothenic acid (B_5) is found in liver, yeast, salmon, vegetables, dairy foods, eggs, grains, and meat.
- B_6 (pyridoxine) is found in potatoes, bananas, raisin bran cereal, lentils, liver, turkey, and tuna.
- B_{12} (cobalamin) is found in dairy foods, eggs, meat, fish, poultry, and seaweed.
- Biotin is found in organ meats, oatmeal, egg yolk, soy, bananas, peanuts, and brewer's yeast.

- Choline is found in liver, soybeans, oatmeal, cabbage, cauliflower, egg yolks, meat, and some vegetables.
- Chromium (a mineral) is found in brewer's yeast, nonrefined grains, and cereals.
- Cysteine (amino acid) is found in most high-protein foods.
- D_3 is found in egg yolks, butter, and vitamin D–fortified foods. (It is also created during a chemical reaction that starts when skin is exposed to sunlight.)
- Folate (folic acid) is found in beans, leafy green vegetables, citrus fruits, beets, wheat germ, and meat.
- Iodine is found in seafood, iodized salt, sea vegetables (for example, kelp).
- Manganese is found in nuts, wheat germ, wheat bran, leafy green vegetables, beet tops, and pineapple.
- Magnesium is found in nuts, grains, beans, dark green vegetables, fish, and meat.
- Molybdenum is found in beans, legumes, dark leafy green vegetables, grains, and hard tap water.

These natural vitamins and minerals particularly promote healthy skin:

- Calcium (a mineral) is found in dairy products, sardines, canned salmon, green leafy vegetables, and tofu.
- Copper (a mineral) is found in seafood, liver, legumes, and green vegetables.
- Niacin (B_3) is found in brewer's yeast, fish, meat, and whole grains.
- Potassium (a mineral) is found in bananas, most other fruits, beans, milk, potatoes, and vegetables.
- Riboflavin (B_2) is found in dairy foods, eggs, meat, leafy green vegetables, and enriched grains.
- Selenium (a mineral) is found in Brazil nuts, yeast, whole grains, and seafood.
- Sulfur (a mineral) is found in fish, eggs, and meat.
- Thiamin (B_1) is found in wheat germ, whole wheat, peas, beans, enriched flour, fish, peanuts, and meat.
- Vitamin A is found in liver, dairy products, vegetables, and cod liver oil.

- Vitamin C (ascorbic acid) is found in broccoli, red peppers, currants, brussels sprouts, parsley, rose hips, acerola berries, citrus fruit, and strawberries.
- Vitamin E (tocopherol) is found in wheat germ oil, nuts, seeds, vegetable oils, whole grains and egg yolks, leafy green vegetables, and soybeans.
- Zinc (a mineral) is found in oysters, meats, eggs, seafood, black-eyed peas, tofu, and wheat germ.

Vitamins and Food Supplements

Vitamins and food supplements can never take the place of the nutrition found in a balanced diet. The medical and nutrition community are divided regarding the usage, dosage, and need for supplements.

Consult a dietitian, nutrition adviser, and your medical internist for the best plan of action to ensure good health and beautiful skin. For instance, there are healthful enhancement amino acids such as cysteine; vitamins A, B, B complex, and PABA; and the minerals zinc and selenium, which combined in the right dosages can help retard the aging process.

The following vitamin therapy is recommended by a well-known family practitioner who I have known for many years who treats skin conditions nutritionally, as well as with medication. He believes that prescription drugs should only be used as a last resort. This is his formula for the healthy adult over thirty years of age. Remember: always check with your physician before taking anything more than an approved over-the-counter supplement.

The doctor recommends this formula as a supplement to a healthy diet and says that it is excellent for more than just your skin. However, I repeat: no diet or health program should begin without a thorough medical checkup first by a licensed physician. The doctor's formula meets the minimum needs, indicated by the latest research, as

RECOMMENDED NUTRIENT THERAPY FOR DAILY INTAKE	
VITAMIN AND MINERAL NUTRIENTS	**QUANTITY**
Vitamin A (60% beta-carotene)	25,000 I.U.
Vitamin C	1,200 mg
Vitamin D_3	100 I.U.
Vitamin E	400 I.U.
Thiamin	100 mg
Riboflavin	50 mg
Niacin niacinamide	190 mg
Vitamin B_6	100 mg
Folate	800 mcg
Vitamin B_{12}	100 mcg
Biotin	300 mcg
Pantothenic acid	500 mg
Iodine	200 mcg
Magnesium	500 mg
Zinc	25 mg
Selenium	200 mcg
Manganese	20 mg
Chromium	200 mcg
Molybdenum	100 mcg
Potassium	99 mg
Calcium	500 mg

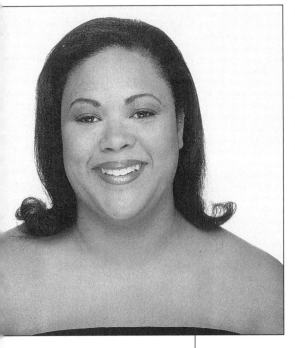

appropriate for enhancing your health and retarding the aging process.

HEALTH AND WEIGHT

The American Dietetic Association and the U.S. Department of Health and Human Services publish dietary guidelines for adult men and women, and of course, you must consult your primary health provider if you are underweight or overweight. Your ideal weight, based upon your height, sex, and age are important factors to consider when making dietary choices. Some of us burn fat at a faster rate than others do. Your nutrition needs are determined by the rate at which you burn fat. (Men usually need between 2,200 and 2,800 calories each day; women require only 1,500 to 2,400.)

When you select foods that are high in fat, sodium, and sugar, you increase your risk of heart attack, stroke, diabetes, and having high cholesterol levels and high blood pressure.

EATING RIGHT AND THE EVENING OUT

Here are some eating tips to help you enjoy a night on the town:

TIPS FOR RESTAURANT DINING

- Try to order easily recognized foods. That way, you'll be able to estimate their fat, sodium, and sugar content. If you're not sure about the caloric count in a dish, ask.

- If you feel that you should "feast" when you dine out, select extra vegetables, salad, and vegetable juices for your meal, rather than extra starches or carbohydrates.

- Restaurant portions are much larger than normal portions. Plan to share your meal with a friend or bring home leftovers for lunch the next day. Pigging out is so 1990s.

- Do not skip meals. To develop better eating habits, consume smaller portions, for good health and better skin.

Now let me give you some "don'ts" and "dos" for healthier black skin. (I place the "don'ts" first here because they can undo all of the "dos.")

Calorie Count on the Web

Get current on specified foods and the breakdown on the calories you burn in given exercises in order to maintain a daily log of weight maintenance activities.

—cyberdiet.com

Remember: the effects of these bad habits are more noticeable on black skin than on white, whereas the good habits are helpful for everyone.

Dos and *Don'ts* for Healthier Skin

●   *Don'ts*

1. Don't smoke. Smoking cuts down on the amount of oxygen getting to the tissues, resulting in impaired circulation and a breakdown or preaging of skin tissue. The results are dry lips, lines and wrinkles, dull ashy complexion, and sagging skin. Nicotine is a toxic substance—a poison.

2. Don't consume excessive amounts of caffeine. Usually you think of caffeine as primarily being in coffee and tea; however, sodas are the greater culprits. Caffeine increases stress and can be diuretic, which means it takes water from your system. This results in more work for your kidney and bladder organs, which can show on the face.

3. Don't sunburn. Ultraviolet rays from the sun dry out the skin. The deeper the tan, the deeper the moisture loss. Dry skin loses its flexibility, softness, and suppleness, giving a dry preaged look. Without sufficient moisture the skin will line and wrinkle. Even creams can only do so much good. It may take years to see the damage, but once done it is just about irreversible.

4. Don't drink alcohol. Those who consistently drink too much decrease their food and water intake, resulting in improper nutrition from a lack of vitamins and minerals—especially B_1, which is necessary for healthy skin. Just one or two cocktails or glasses of wine a day can dehydrate tissues and make wrinkles more prominent.

5. Don't take too many or long baths in the winter. Long baths in the winter remove the protective oils from the skin, which are helping to keep the necessary skin moisture in the cells for suppleness. Once the oils are removed, moisture is drawn off. Even bath oils are not

STOP!
Smoking Can Change Your Life!

Eyes:	You'll have fewer lines and wrinkles.
Nose:	Sinus congestion will subside.
Heart:	Heart conditions will decrease.
Mouth:	Healthy gums reappear. Teeth become bright and breath fresher.
Tongue:	The taste of food improves.
Throat:	Smoker's cough disappears.
Lungs:	Lung function will increase.
Hands:	Tobacco stains will disappear.
Contact:	The American Cancer Society, locally or on the Internet at www.cancer.org.

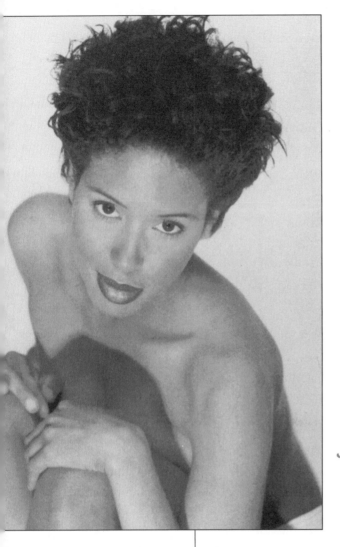

as effective as your natural oils, but do use them and moisture lotions, sprays, and body splash after a bath.

6. Don't use pure petroleum jelly and its by-products, cocoa butter sticks, or oil as a facial skin moisturizer, if it is not water soluble. Oils are not moisturizers and will not make your skin soft and supple. They will hold existing moisture in, but unfortunately the oils, if heavy or thick, can clog the pores, causing eruptions. Oils will definitely cause a shine, often giving a false impression of oily skin when in fact the skin may be dry. This is particularly true for those who are swarthy or dark-complexioned.

7. Don't leave makeup on overnight. If makeup is left on too long, it can irritate skin, clog pores, and cause eruptions.

8. Don't stay in overheated rooms unless absolutely necessary. Overheated rooms usually are dry and will draw the moisture from your skin, helping dry it out.

9. Don't overeat. Being overweight is unhealthy and affects the condition of your skin. The stored fat accumulates peroxides, which are immune-system depressants, leaving the body more open to attack, including allergies. An unhealthy body affects the long-range quality of your skin, particularly the dermis.

Dos

1. Do exercise. Proper exercise causes perspiration, which cleanses the pores and removes impurities from your system. It also increases blood flow, bringing needed nutrients to the surface. Ten minutes of peak exercise a day can be healthful and effective.

2. Do drink six to eight glasses of water daily. Your system (vital organs) needs water; your cells need water to replace lost water and maintain skin moisture.

3. Do use a water filter. You should drink nonchlorinated, nonmetal-ionized water. These are oxidants, which bring on preaging symptoms. Use a filter that draws off these minerals and trace elements from your water. Filters are cheaper in the long run than bottled water and provide water that is equally palatable. Your cooking and ice cube water should be as pure as your drinking water.

4. Do have a full-length mirror in your bedroom. Make sure you face the mirror nude, from all angles. This will either help keep you on your diet as you see the positive changes or it will help you get on a diet if you don't like the additional poundage.

5. Do use nutrient supplements if you drink alcohol. I mentioned the loss of vitamin B_1 and resultant poor diet that usually accompany excessive drinking. This suggestion is not to be taken as a tacit approval of drinking alcohol. But I'm aware that many may not stop drinking alcohol and yet will want some type of

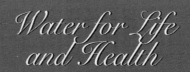

Water for Life and Health

YOUR WATER WORKOUT

■ Health clubs nationwide are adding and improving water fitness and exercise programs. Both young and mature adults find that exercising in water is less stressful on the body.

■ Water aerobics, yoga, aquatic kicking, water walking, and running exercises offer the following benefits:

> stretching
>
> aerobic conditioning
>
> flexibility
>
> strength conditioning
>
> relaxed muscles and joints
>
> naturally ridding the body of excess water and fat

Beauty Tip: Water exercises are becoming more popular because there is less stress to joints and lower risk of injury.

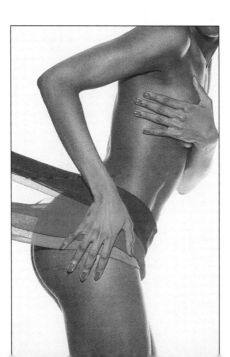

RECOMMENDED NUTRITIONAL SUPPLEMENTS FOR DRINKERS

The following nutritional supplements are recommended for moderate drinkers, who might have an occasional glass of wine. It was prepared by Durk Pearson and Sandy Shaw, authors of *Life Extension.* They list the total dose per day, to be divided into three doses and taken with meals:

SUPPLEMENT	QUANTITY
Vitamin A	1,200 I.U.
Vitamin B	.12 g
Vitamin B_2	24 mg
Vitamin B_3 (niacin)	72 mg
Vitamin B_5	24 mg
Vitamin B_6	60 mg
Vitamin B_{12}	60 mcg
Vitamin C	.36 g
Vitamin E	120 I.U.
Choline	.36 g
Cysteine (not crystal)	.24 g
Zinc (chelated)	60 mg
Selenium	30 mcg

Consult your physician before starting such a program, and do not follow this formula if you are diabetic, suffer from ulcers, or drink heavily.

protection. See Recommended Nutritional Supplements for Drinkers for recommendations.

6.   Do eat properly. In addition to eating healthful meals, you can take vitamin, mineral, and amino acid supplements. Certainly a vegetarian diet with nutrition supplements is healthful and produces healthy skin, but as a general rule, eat raw and steamed vegetables, fish, and chicken. Limit your intake of red meat; candy, desserts, and sugar in general; tea and coffee; and sodas. Take cod liver oil, zinc, vitamins C and E, and lecithin.

7.   Do weigh yourself regularly. Every week, get on the same scale in the same room at the same time.

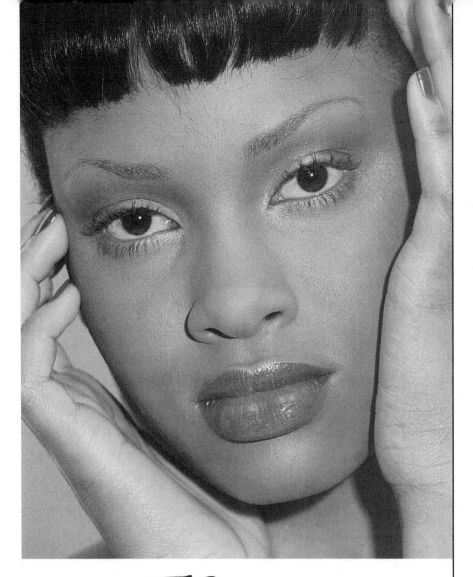

HOW TO TOUCH
YOUR FACE

3

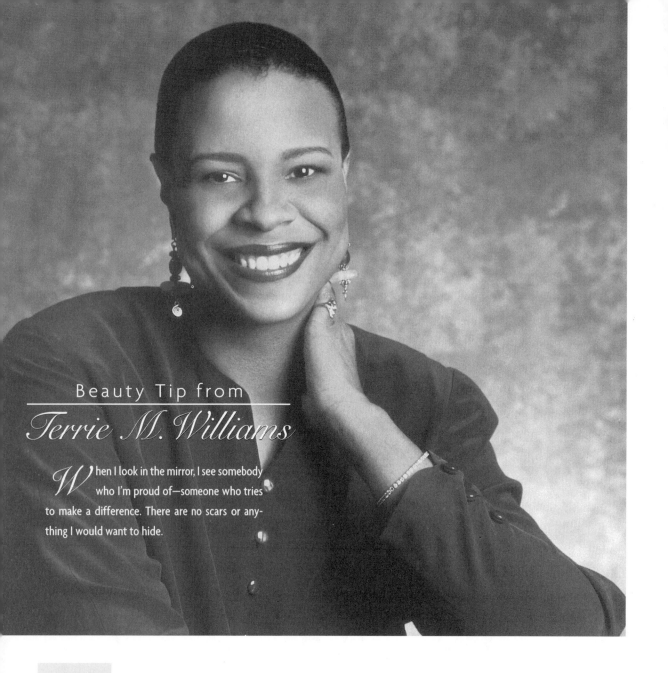

Terrie M. Williams

*W*hen I look in the mirror, I see somebody
who I'm proud of—someone who tries
to make a difference. There are no scars or anything I would want to hide.

Terrie M. Williams, founder and president of The Terrie Williams Agency, is a public relations professional, published author, lecturer, deal maker, and community activist. Terrie, who is one of the country's most highly sought-after speakers, is also the author of *The Personal Touch: What You Really Need to Succeed in Today's Fast-Paced Business World* and *Stay Strong: Simple Life Lessons for Teens.*

$\mathcal{H}ave$ you ever thought about how you touch or should touch your face? If you are like most women, you probably have not. Because I consider how to touch your skin so important, I have made it the first "how to" section in this book. You can use all the correct products and colors, and follow the best nutrition program, but still damage your face because you touch it improperly. By "touching your face," I refer to how you attend to it with your hands, such as when you clean it, apply toner or astringent, or blend on moisturizer and other similar products.

$\mathcal{D}$IRECTED HAND MOVEMENTS

You should try to touch your face only when your hands are clean. Your facial skin has enough to deal with without you accidentally adding dirt and bacteria from your hands. There is a proper technique for touching your face, based on how the muscles and skin on your face are attached and how they work.

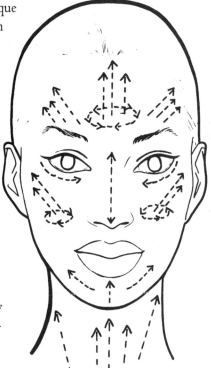

You should always use your fingers in the direction that reduces stress—that works with, rather than against, your facial muscles and skin. The illustration to the right shows the direction your fingers should move on various parts of your neck and face. When cleaning or massaging your neck, move upward with your hands or fingers to the chin line. When touching your face, use your fingertips in a circular motion, moving outward from the nose to the hairline except around the eyes.

Remember: although you have five fingers, they are not equally appropriate for your face. The ring finger is most serviceable. It is your weakest finger; yes, it is even weaker than your little finger. Test it and you will see. You want to use a light touch, so use the ring finger, particularly when working in the eye areas, which have the thinnest layers of epidermal skin. (That is why age lines show themselves faster and more often in these areas.)

THE EYE AREA

When cleansing or massaging your face around the eyes, always work from the outer temple inward toward the bridge of the nose. You should move in this direction because the facial muscles around the eyes are suspended from the temple toward the nose. Going in the opposite direction stretches the skin and muscles, and risks damage. Once damaged, there is little that can be done, other than to have injections of collagen or silicone to fill the damaged area. But because black skin is easily bruised and retains dark spots, most dermatologists are reluctant to have black women take these injections, which could result in either or both of these conditions. I repeat: always use the ring finger under your eyes.

THE REST OF THE FACE

Use the fingertips of your first three fingers for your cheeks, and for your forehead, move in a circular motion out to the hairline. The chin is massaged with the first three fingers of each hand, moving from the center of the chin outward with a gentle, rotating motion.

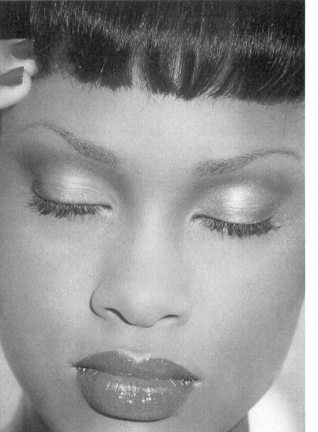

GENTLY STIMULATE AS YOU TOUCH

Whenever you touch your skin, you should try to gently massage it at the same time. The stimulation from gently slapping and massaging the face is very helpful. This form of touching causes the blood to rush upward to the surface, replenishing the skin while drawing away impurities and leaving a nice glow. Another positive result is that this action reduces not only facial stress but stress throughout your body as well. Relaxing the facial muscles may reduce those lines in the forehead and around the mouth or prevent them from getting deeper.

If you have oily skin, however, you should stimulate your skin less often than if you have dry, because frequent massaging will bring additional oil to the surface.

$\mathcal{Y}$OUR SKINCARE AND MAINTENANCE TOOLS

Now that you know how to touch your face, whether you are massaging or cleansing it, you need to learn which cosmetic instruments to use when applying makeup to your face. There are approximately seven tools that most women may use, and we will look at them one at a time: facecloths, buff scrubs, cosmetic cotton balls and pads, loofahs (sponges), facial tissues, cosmetic swabs, and facial brushes.

FACECLOTHS

Most people, including women, use a facecloth to wash their face and body. Unfortunately, many women do not think about the abrasive quality of their facecloth. Many cloths, after being wet from use, will dry and harden overnight, with the cloth's nap turned into a myriad of hard little bristles. When you use this cloth to scrub your face, the results—whether initially visible or not—are that you bruise and often cut the outer layer of skin, particularly around the eyes. So while cleansing, you have abused your skin when your intent was just the opposite.

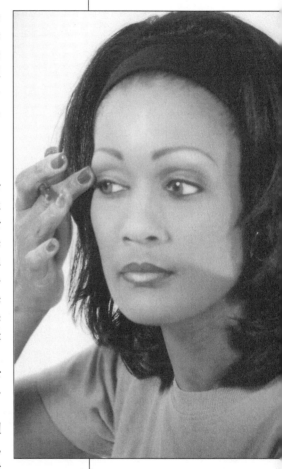

The guiding principle here is to show loving care to your face. Be gentle and kind. Buy and use only pure cotton facecloths because they dry softer and maintain a soft nap.

When you use a cotton facecloth, wrap it around your hand or fingers like a mitten. Work your finger, covered by the cloth, over your face as described earlier. Don't rub hard to stimulate or remove flaky skin. If you want to stimulate your face, use the massaging and slapping technique described. It will not bruise, irritate, or damage your skin or the capillaries below the surface. Don't forget: work the eye area gently, and move the cloth from the temple to the bridge of the nose. Do the forehead with a circular motion, moving outward and upward to the hairline.

One of the leading skincare companies sent me a sample of their cleansing cloths. I've used the cloths with success. They are textured, cleansing, hand glove–type facecloths, which when combined with water, release lathering cleansers and conditioners to remove dirt, oil, and makeup. The specially treated cloths gently exfoliate and smooth the skin's texture.

BUFF SCRUBS

Buff scrubs are made of synthetic materials. They are used in washing, scrubbing, and stimulating the face. I have a general aversion to buff scrubs because black women have to be so careful in using them. All too often, because of their harsh synthetic quality, buff scrubs cut or cause abrasions to the skin, resulting in a burn that may darken and become a spot. If you use a buff scrub to stimulate, you must be extraordinarily careful and use it in the gentlest fashion.

If you use a buff scrub, do it no more than once or twice a week, and then only with kindness and gentleness. Black women with acne should never use buff scrubs.

LOOFAHS

Loofahs, or luffas, are natural sponges, but they are harder and have a straw-like look until they are soaked in water. There are other natural sponges, such as silk sea sponges, which are very soft and can be used for applying makeup. When choosing a loofah, buy the softest and least abrasive one you can find. There is no doubt that, after use, your face will have a radiant glow and the look of good health, but this could be deceiving. It is possible that the abrasive quality of even a soft loofah may irritate the skin in the process of stimulating the blood flow. It is best suited for using on your skin from the neck down.

Before using, always thoroughly soak the loofah in water, so it is as soft as possible. If necessary, err on the side of caution. When your face is at risk, don't use a loofah regularly; reserve it for special occasions, and then use it gently.

FACIAL TISSUES

There are two major "don'ts" when you think of using facial tissues on your face. The first is that you don't use tissues that contain wood pulp. Tissues applied to the face should be soft. When wood pulp touches your face, it can cut, scratch, or split the delicate skin mantle without your feeling or immediately knowing it. This damage can result in bruising or darkening of the healed scratch, and can even develop into a keloid (thickening of scar tissue). Generally, the more expensive tissues are free of wood pulp.

The second precaution is that you don't use tissues if you have excessive facial hair, skin eruptions, and so on. The fibers of the tissue may cling or get into skin openings, causing infections, discomfort, and additional problems. What is most interesting is that these concerns probably seem unnecessary because you may think they haven't happened to you. Unfortunately, the damage generally is not visible, unless you really look for it. This is similar to the damage caused by smoking in that the injury to your body is not seen initially. But by the time it is, the damage has been done.

As I consistently plead, err on the side of caution. You have everything to gain and nothing to lose. When working with tissues, use them gently and use only those free of wood fiber, and when your face is smooth and free of pimples, bumps, and other blemishes. There is good news though. Most moisture tissues are soft, irritant free, and have no wood fibers.

COTTON BALLS AND PADS

When using cotton balls and pads, think of them as if they were tissues. The same potential problems from using facial tissues exist for cotton balls and pads. Buy only the pure natural-fiber balls and pads and avoid synthetic cosmetic "cotton." How can they be man-made and still be cotton? They cannot. They are damaging to your skin, so be careful; check them out.

Real cotton balls and pads are excellent because they are sanitary. You use one, throw it away, and get another. Cotton balls and pads are particularly good for applying toners, astringents, and fresheners, or in cleansing the delicate tissue around the eye.

COSMETIC SWABS

Your swabs should be of the best brands and of pure cotton, spun properly so that the fine cotton hairs are intact and flat on the head of the swab. This is important because loose fine cotton hairs can damage the skin, particularly when the swabs are used to clean the corners of the eyes. Properly designed pure cotton swabs, either round or flat, are excellent for applying eye shadow, color, and for cleansing around the nose and under the eyes. Again, as you use them in these areas, make sure that you work from the temple inward toward the bridge of the nose.

I must mention here that swabs should be used in the outer ear and not placed in the ear canal. I know this point does not relate to your face, but always when I am interviewed or on tour, women mention using swabs for their ears as well as their face. There are better ways to clean your ear canal than to place a swab in it.

FACIAL BRUSHES

I like most of the brushes on the market today, and I consider them equal in value to pure cotton facecloths for facial use. I am particularly fond of brushes made of gentle natural or man-made fibers. Some are sponge types while others have very soft bristles. The one type that I recommend black women avoid is the rubber facial brush. Black skin bruises and marks easily, and a rubber facial brush may cause a friction burn, resulting in a bruise and discoloration.

THE BEST TOOL FOR EACH JOB

Despite all of the tools mentioned above, the tools you should always feel safe using on your face are your own clean fingers. You can control them better than any of these other cosmetics tools. Next best are the natural cotton facecloths and facial brush, excluding the rubber bristled ones. Don't forget: when using a facecloth, wrap it around your fingers so that you are using your fingers as though they were inside a cotton mitten. When using a facial brush, be gentle and use the same motion you would if you were using only your fingers.

Tissues, and cotton balls, and cotton pads and swabs should all be made of pure cotton. Swabs and balls are for limited service: swabs for under the eyes and in crevices around the nose; cotton balls for applying toners, astringents, and fresheners, and for cleansing. Tissues have the most limited use, mainly for cleaning or toning the face. Yet all these cosmetic tools can be serviceable if they are of fine quality and are used with care.

DON'T FORGET

1. Use the fingers, and particularly the ring finger, when cleansing or touching the face.
2. The ring finger should be used in the eye area, and the movement should be from the temple toward the bridge of the nose.

3. Finger motion should be circular and outward to the hairline except for under the eyes.

4. Fingers on the neck should move upward to the chin line.

5. When stimulating the face, use the fingertips with a gentle slapping or patting motion in the directions outlined.

6. Wrap your pure cotton facecloth around your fingers and touch your face for cleansing as though your fingers were in a cotton mitten.

7. The same movements you employ in using a facecloth should be used when working with a facial brush (not rubber).

YOUR DAILY BEAUTY HABIT RESOLUTIONS

- Water. Water. Water. Drink at least seven to eight glasses per day.
- Eat with your skin beauty in mind—avoid fried foods and eat fewer fats. Remember, each fresh vegetables and more fruits.
- Maintain body conditioning for muscle toning and shaping.
- Get adequate sleep—at least eight hours. It brings peace of mind and allows the body to regenerate. (Take one hour to just rest and breathe deeply in a room with some ventilation and a humidifier. Relax with a warm cup of decaf tea, hot chocolate, water with a slice of lemon, or tomato juice.) Sleep and rest are as important as water for better-looking skin.
- Try eye and lip moisture replacement during the evening restful hours. It allows for deep conditioning penetration under and around the eyes and the concave grooves of the lips.
- Be sure to use a moisturizer for your skin type when commuting on poorly ventilated suburban trains and traveling in pressurized airplane cabins.

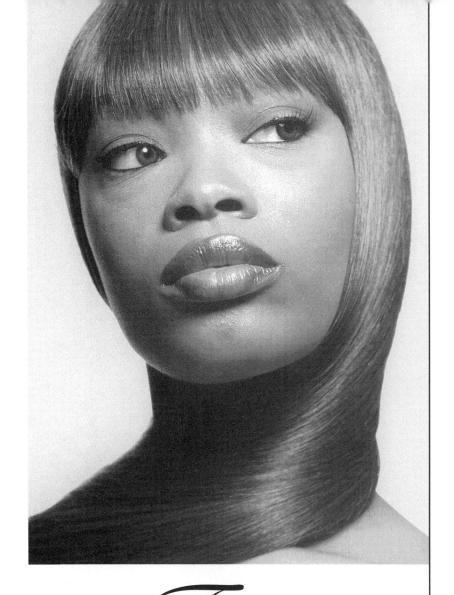

FACIAL HAIR, BLEMISHES, AND OTHER FACIAL CONDITIONS

4

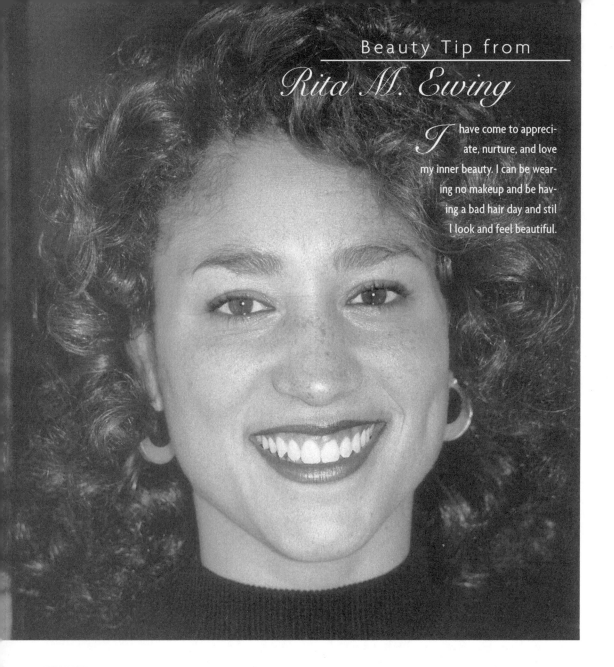

Beauty Tip from
Rita M. Ewing

I have come to appreciate, nurture, and love my inner beauty. I can be wearing no makeup and be having a bad hair day and still I look and feel beautiful.

R Rita M. Ewing, wife of basketball legend Patrick Ewing, is the founder of One-on-One Management, which teaches home office management techniques to professional athletes. She also coauthored the novel *Homecourt Advantage,* and is a partner in the Hue-Man bookstore based in Harlem, New York.

In this chapter I explain how certain skin features develop, such as facial hair, freckles, pimples and blemishes, blackheads and white-heads, age spots, and so on. If you understand what causes these conditions and know how to cover or remove them effectively and safely, then you will feel better about your face and about yourself.

Facial Hair

Removing facial hair is a concern for many women, especially black women. Black women do not necessarily have more facial or body hair than white women, but the problem has to be approached differently. In beauty salons and clinics, I constantly see black women attacking the hair on their face, underarms, and legs. These women buy product after product at cosmetics counters in discount drug chains and department stores. Personally, I don't see facial hair on women as being a problem. But our society has made it a problem. In North America, facial hair is not considered to be an attractive feature or part of female beauty.

There are places in the world where men find the hair on women sexy, but this chapter is not for those men or women. Our society sees facial hair as a problem—for example, when hair bumps detract from one's appearance or interfere with makeup application.

Facial Waxing

Areas of concern are usually the facial hair at the temples, hair at the jaw-line moving back toward the earlobe, and hair on the upper lip or chin. More women than you might realize have thick hair growing above their upper lip or on the base of their chin. If you want clear skin, then such hair must be removed, especially if you wish your makeup to have a clear, smooth appearance.

Fair-skinned women with blonde or sandy-colored hair can readily bleach unwanted facial hairs and make the hairs appear to fade or become translucent. For most black women, bleaching is not an option. The bleached hair stands out prominently against your dark skin. The only recourse is to have this facial hair professionally removed by waxing. Waxing is a hair-removal technique that involves applying a paste of warm wax to the hair surface. The wax is allowed to dry, then it is stripped away. As it is stripped away, so is the hair, leaving the skin beneath smooth. It is painless, and the method can keep the area free of hair for three to six weeks. Another option is to purchase an over-the-counter hair-removing wax product from a drugstore chain or department store. You can use these products at home, and while the process takes time, you will save money. The home method keeps hairs off for nearly six weeks.

Electrolysis and Depilatory Techniques

Hair can be removed permanently through electrolysis or depilatrom; the latter is a popular new treatment. Sometimes you may experience a degree of sensitivity from depilatrom, but this doesn't last long. Electrolysis, however, can be very costly, since you pay by the number of hairs removed.

Some dermatologists do not recommend electrolysis for black women because many develop scarring around the pores. These areas are damaged and become unsightly after the hairs have been pulled through or by them. Some women build up so much scar tissue around the pores that they develop keloids (bumps composed of scar tissue). Black skin, although many layered, is susceptible to scarring—certainly more so than white skin. If you choose electrolysis, make sure you go to a competent electrolysis technician who understands black skin.

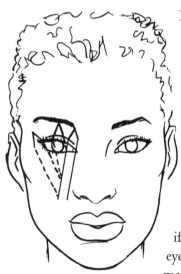

To determine the best length and thickness of your brow, hold your eyebrow pencil to each nostril and straight up along the nose to the eyebrow. Where it touches the eyebrow is where the brow should begin. Hair between the eyebrows should be removed. Position the pencil vertically over the center of your eye to the beginning of the arch. When you position the pencil from the nose to the outer edge of the eye, you determine the endpoint of the brow and arch.

There are modern techniques that enable you to remove hair, so you can effectively do hair-removal procedures at home yourself. Usually such items are sold in the beauty appliance section of a retail cosmetics outlet or the cosmetics counter in better drugstores.

Unruly Eyebrows

Another area of unwanted hair growth on the face is the eyebrows. Knowing the technique of shaping the eyebrows is important. A woman is considered lucky if she has eyebrow hairs that lay flat and eyebrows that are well shaped to complement her eyes. However, most women are not so lucky, and they have to have some hairs removed to get a nice look. Many women prefer not to wear a great deal of eye shadow for good reason. Bushy or unruly hairs springing through their eye shadow and highlighter would be unsightly. Others have eyebrow hairs removed because they don't like the way their eyebrows look and can't find a way to manage them. For example, bushy or heavy and coarse eyebrows may require some plucking.

I find it most unattractive when a woman shaves off her eyebrows and then uses an eyebrow pencil to draw in a line. This gives the face a severe look. Why shave the eyebrow off and then put a new one on, instead of properly shaping or filling in your existing eyebrow?

Nothing is more unsightly than a dramatic, overplucked eyebrow either. The problem that this may cause—beyond unsightliness—is that when you continually pluck hairs in certain spots, you pull out some of the roots and the hairs will never grow back. Thus you are left with a patchy-looking brow.

Look in the mirror and honestly assess the length and thickness of your brows. If they are bushy and are overpowering your face, then you should remove some hairs. If your eyebrows are too thick and spotty with nicks, then you should shape the brow to complement a natural eyeline. With a brow pencil, you can stroke in between the spaces, filling and shaping the brow. The drawn-on pencil look is out of fashion; instead, start from the center of the eye and go upward to the temple, removing from eight to ten hairs.

Tweeze the stray hairs underneath your brow also. The ideal eyebrow arch is smooth and soft—often referred to as a moon shape. Shape your eyebrow with the

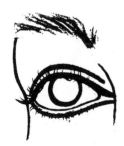

peak at the center of the brow. To check or correct the shape of your eyebrows, see the preceding illustration.

Many of you have written to me about the clean, sleek look around the eyes that the celebrities are wearing. This sleek look including the eyes, eyebrows, and lips has grown in popularity and appeal during the past seasons.

Beauty tip: if you are not sure about shaping, then take a pencil lighter or darker than the brow hairs and draw in lightly your desired new shape for comparison. (See chapter 17 on eyes for more details.)

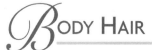

BODY HAIR

You may want to remove hair from your legs, around the neck, and under your arms. Waxing can rid these areas of unwanted hair. There are also depilatories sold in any beauty department that easily whisk away the hair. Let the depilatory set for a few moments and then wipe or rinse hair off with water. Always apply a moisturizer after removing hair from either the face or lower body parts.

SKIN PROBLEMS

Let's look at the skin "problems" most black women ask me about. Remember, even if you avoid the "don'ts" and do the "dos" in chapters 7 through 10, you may still have skin problems.

BREAKING OUT

There is no one specific cause for "breaking out," but it can almost always be stopped or controlled. No matter what the cause, good, regular skincare can help. A healthy regimen plus internal medicine can cure most, if not all, incidents of breaking out and prevent their recurrence.

A physician should determine the type, form, and amount of medicine you need. Obviously, you need not go to the doctor for every blemish. But when you have a blemish that doesn't go away and it bothers you, seek medical advice. Yes, even acne is a condition worthy of a doctor's visit. The person at the cosmetics counter is a beauty adviser, not a physician, even if he or she is a licensed cosmetologist.

The Pill Is Not a Skin Enhancer

Many women have asked me about taking birth control pills to clear up their skin problems. At this time there is no consensus on the pill's effectiveness in treating skin problems. Research has been done in this area, but at least 25 percent of those studied have seen their skin worsen, and the largest group studied saw no change in skin condition at all. The estrogen in birth control pills is sometimes used as a skin treatment, but I am opposed to using the pill that way. There are possible side effects from birth control pills, among them an increase in skin pigmentation, and for some women, the skin gets mottled and darkish.

Menses and Skin Eruptions

Yes, there is an established relationship between your periods and facial eruptions or breakouts. But preventive medication is available. Don't forget, though, that carefully cleansing your face before, during, and after your period definitely helps.

Blemishes

Blemishes are skin faults—for example, blackheads, whiteheads, and pimples. You should never probe and squeeze a blackhead. Squeezing a blackhead can damage the surrounding areas, and you can spread the infection to below the surface, causing other places on your face to erupt. The best way to remove or eliminate blackheads is to keep your skin clean. Remember, you can't have a blackhead without a clogged, oily pore. Therefore, the best approach is super cleanliness—morning and night, and sometimes in between.

The whitehead is so named because the head of the eruption is whitish in color. In stubborn cases when whiteheads persist, you should see a doctor or dermatologist, who'll treat them with a miniature scalpel or electric needle. Whiteheads found around the eye (milia) are generally believed to be caused by abrasions or small cuts.

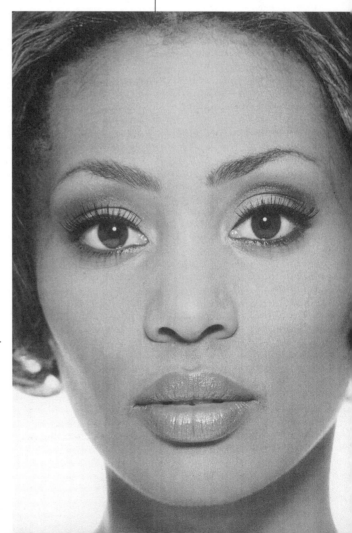

BLOTCHES

To avoid blotches, avoid excessive sunlight. Limit the amount of ultraviolet light that hits your face by using a sunblock, either all over the face or on just the mottled area. Actually, sunblock is a great base for makeup. If mottled, darkish spots already exist on your face, it is possible to have then removed through dermabrasion—the wearing down of the skin layers until there is clear skin. There are also abrasive scrubs and bleaching creams that can be used directly on the affected area that help work off the dead, darkened skin.

WRINKLES AND SAGGING SKIN

Wrinkles and sagging skin are due to a breakdown of the skin's collagen, connective tissue that maintains the skin's elasticity and tightness. Proper skincare not only keeps your skin clear and free of blemishes, but also retards the breaking down of the skin's collagen, reducing wrinkles and sagging skin. Therefore, it is critical that you maintain an adequate collagen level. This can easily be attained by consuming adequate amounts of vitamin C daily. A natural source of vitamin C is rose hips. A rich natural source of

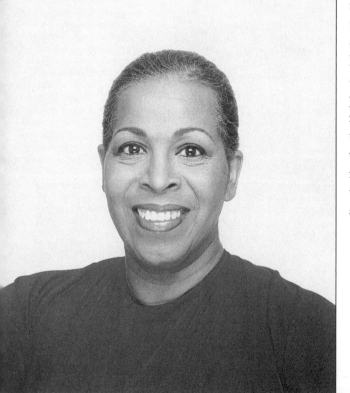

vitamins, rose hips contain twenty to forty times more vitamin C than oranges. They also have twenty-five times more vitamin A, 28 percent more calcium, and 25 percent more iron than oranges. Rose hips are extremely rich in bioflavonoids—cofactors in the vitamin C complex. But whatever you take—natural foods or vitamins—make vitamin C one of your staples, for it is a most important health and facial rejuvenation vitamin. By utilizing these nutritional tips, you are helping to retard the aging process and collagen breakdown, which will help you maintain more youthful-looking skin while improving your overall health.

$\mathcal{S}$KINCARE AND SUN EXPOSURE

Black women, men, and children are spending more time in the sun—on cruise ships, sunning, swimming in tropical countries, on honeymoons, or just touring. And we're also visiting relatives for homecomings and having barbecues and beach parties in the sun, not to mention playing golf, tennis, and other sports.

WHAT YOU SHOULD KNOW ABOUT SUN PRODUCTS

The FDA has put together guidelines for the cosmetic industry to measure and rate how long we can stay in the sun without burning and damaging our skin, which can lead to skin surface cancer and premature aging. The industry supports 15 to 30 SPF (sun protection factor) as recommended protection for the skin. I am not a medical person, and I certainly recommend that you consult your primary health-care provider to determine the appropriate product to meet your needs (even for over-the-counter sun products). When the sun is most intense, between noon and 3 P.M., in most African and Caribbean countries there is little movement outside. People who must be out in the sun wear beautiful multicolored reflecting garments for optimum protection. (These are made from patented registered fabrics that are woven in a way that protects people from the sun.) In Latin American countries, men and women for centuries have worn the wide hats (sombreros) to block the damaging rays of the sun. Here in the United States, where we bare all, some type of sunscreen and sunblock skin-conditioning care is necessary for protection.

Cosmetics companies include sunscreen ingredients in their moisturizers and skincare products. Be sure your eye moisture product is free of irritants and fragrances.

Sunscreen formulas come in gels, creams, and liquid sprays, and are nongreasy and long lasting. Formulations with zinc titanium dioxide or zinc oxide block and reflect the sunlight away from the face and body and are best for long exposure to the sun.

SUN OBSERVATIONS

Dark-complexioned people of color often cannot identify sunburned, overexposed, damaged skin. The dark skin takes on a bluish aura and is very sensitive to the touch. It can become painful and infected if not treated. More

SUNSCREEN
Beauty
T·I·P·S

- When moving about during the work week, wear a hat that blocks direct sun rays and sunglasses that provide protection from harmful ultraviolet A and B rays.
- Speaking in general, most of us have full lips. Lips need protection too. More men are also using lip-care protection formulas in winter and summer. (Ask your beauty adviser, or read the labels yourself, to find out if lip moisturizers, lip balm, lipstick, and lip glosses have SPF 25 or 30).
- When you are active in the sun and it's hot and the humidity is high, you sweat more. Remember to reapply sunscreen protection and drink liquids.
- After you shower and towel off, you must reapply moisture and sunscreen protection.
- Before and after swimming in a pool or at the beach, facial and body skin should be reconditioned with sunscreens.

sun exposure under these conditions can make you nauseated and sick, and could lead to skin cancer. Consult a medical internist immediately.

If you develop allergic reactions to either sunscreen or sunblock products, consult a physician immediately.

Your ears, nose, lips, hands, and feet should be protected along with your face and body.

People with acne can benefit from water-soluble gels that can be removed easily without disturbing the problem skin condition. Consult your dermatologist for over-the-counter products.

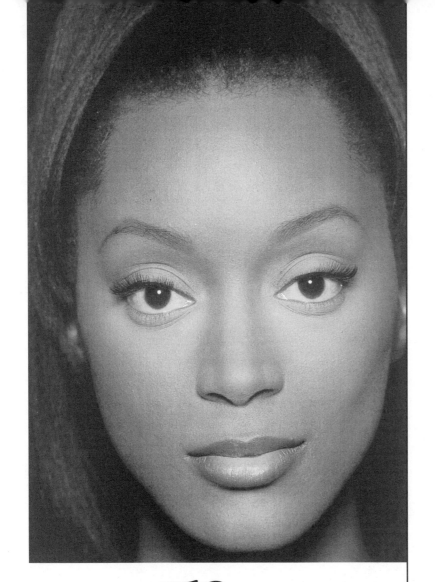

KNOW YOUR SKIN TYPE

5

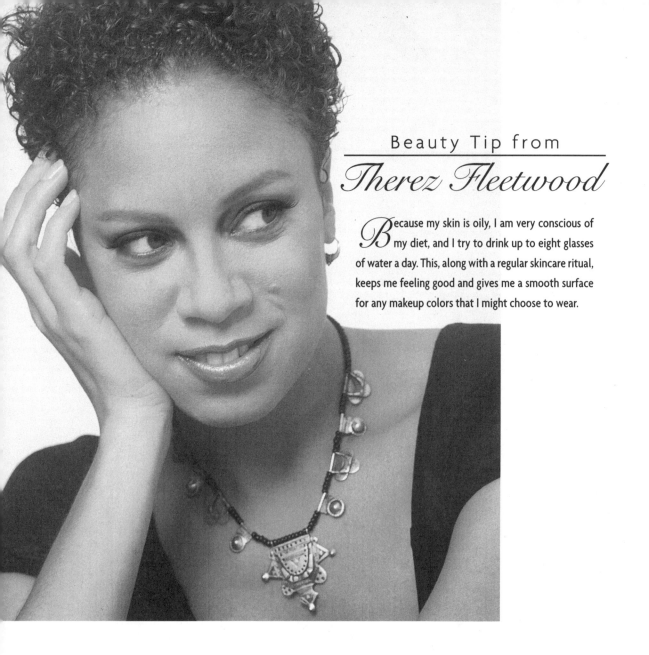

Therez Fleetwood

Because my skin is oily, I am very conscious of my diet, and I try to drink up to eight glasses of water a day. This, along with a regular skincare ritual, keeps me feeling good and gives me a smooth surface for any makeup colors that I might choose to wear.

Therez Fleetwood, one the country's leading designers, has created the award-winning Therez Fleetwood Bridal Wear Collection, which uniquely combines African fabrics, trims, and influences with European cuts and silhouettes. Her designs have been featured in countless magazines, textbooks, and national television programs. Therez is also the author of *The Afrocentric Bride—A Style Guide for the African-American Woman*.

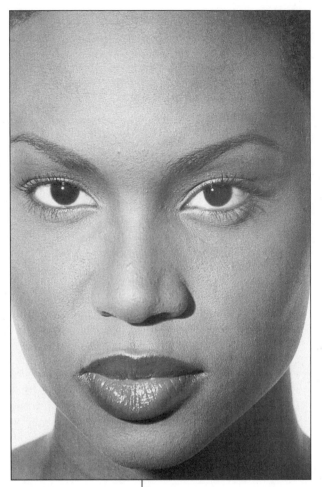

This is my third beauty book for adult African American women. A fourth publication is currently being released for teenagers of color. I have taught famous makeup artists, household consumers, and professional women and men of all careers to be more educated and knowledgeable about purchasing cosmetics that meet their income levels and facial needs. Up to this point, I have worked with you on how to touch your face and what materials to use when cleansing, toning, and stimulating your face. You may be thinking, That's fine. But what do I cleanse or wash my face with? Soap, creams, cleansing lotions, gels, or cleansing cloths?

Before I can help you choose the right type of product to put on your face, you need to determine your skin type. You have to organize what you know about your face in order to become an effective cosmetic consumer, in terms of what is both the best value for your money and is correct for your skin. Remember: what you put on your face can hurt you.

This chapter has three parts. The first helps you determine your skin type. The second discusses appropriate products for your skin type. The third applies the information discussed in chapter 6 to help you use the right products on your face. When you finish this chapter, you will know all the basics for using the methods described throughout this book.

*D*ETERMINING YOUR SKIN TYPE

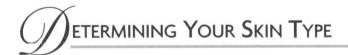

A black woman can have more than one skin type. For instance, you may have a basic skin type that is altered by outside factors. Many women find that there are seasonal or other reasons for their skin type to change. Their skin may become dryer or oilier, or may be more sensitive than usual, based on whether it is spring/summer or fall/winter. Some women find that they have skin changes based on their menstrual period or as a result of dieting, consuming alcohol, taking birth control pills, and even smoking. Additionally, drug abuse, allergies, and aging can affect your skin condition.

These effects are particularly noticeable on black skin because black skin is deceptive—beautifully so, but deceptive. The amount of melanin and carotene in black skin will often cause light to reflect off it, or appear to, rather than to be absorbed, as it is on much lighter skins or on white skin. If there is any perspiration on the nose or chin, the center of a black face may appear shiny. This shiny quality gives the impression that the skin is oily, when actually it may not be. In fact, the skin could be dry.

A Few Rules

You may notice light reflecting off the T-zone as you look in the mirror. (The T-zone is the area of your face that goes across your forehead from temple to temple and down through your nose to your chin.) Look to the left and then to the right of the T-zone, and compare how your skin looks. See if there is a different amount of light reflected on the left and right sides of the T-zone, compared to the T-zone itself.

If the sides of your face and the T-zone are the same, with clean hands touch first your forehead, then the tip of your nose and your chin. If there's perspiration, wipe it away. Though you still need to do more testing, you probably have normal skin. If you feel oil, touch the sides of your face; if they also feel oily, then your skin is oily.

When you look at your face, note any areas that appear different, either patchy, rough, or discolored. Patchiness and roughness are often signs of dry skin; however, your face could have areas that are dry and others that are normal or oily. And this situation can change with the seasons, your health, and possibly with pregnancy.

Clear Your Mind and Clear Your Face

This technique for determining your skin type may seem complex, but I want you to rid yourself of all those old and untrue beliefs you may have had about your skin type. I want you to realize that skin classification requires close attention to your face as well as other conditions affecting your body. I want you to forget the notion that all you have to do is look to the T-zone or type your skin once and the job is done forever.

Thinking that they have sensitive skin because their faces break out, many women buy the wrong products for their faces. This is wasted money and keeps a skin problem unresolved.

CHECK YOUR SKIN TYPE TWICE A YEAR

Evaluate your skin type twice a year: once during spring/summer and once during fall/winter. But don't do it at the very beginning or end of these seasons. Do it a few weeks into each time, and use common sense. If the change in season is very abrupt, evaluate your face sooner; if the change is almost imperceptible, do it a little later. When you change your clothes for the season, that is when to make your test. Of course, I don't mean when you change clothes to be fashionable. I mean when you change for body comfort.

THE SKIN-TYPING QUESTIONNAIRE

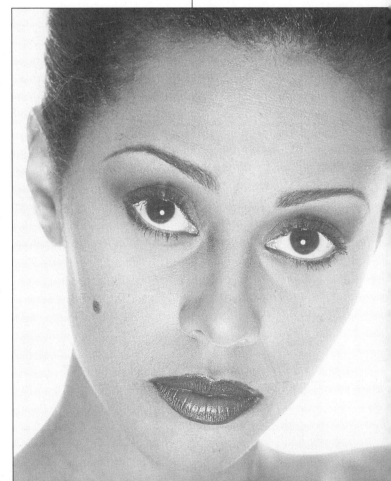

Here is the easy part, which helps take the guesswork and confusion out of typing your skin. I have developed ten questions, the answers to which will help you determine what kind of skin you have. The charts on the following pages show these questions, with characteristics listed for four skin types: oily, combination, dry, and sensitive. Your answers to these ten questions can be matched to the corresponding characteristics. In some instances, there is only one description; in others, two or more situations characterize that skin type.

Remember, I have deliberately given up to four possible skin types. This is to force you to think in terms of that which is most usual, most noticeable.

QUESTIONS TO DETERMINE YOUR SKIN TYPE

QUESTION	OILY
1. Before and after cleansing, can you see oil?	Always
2. Does your skin feel greasy or slick?	T-zone All over
3. If you bathe with deodorant soap, how does your face and body skin feel after an hour, without any type of moisturizer?	Oily forehead, eyelids, nose, and chin
4. What do your pores look like?	Wide, enlarged all over
5. Do you have blackheads or whiteheads?	Many Summer problems
6. Do you break out?	Frequently
7. Do you peel or crack around the forehead, eyes, nose, mouth, lips, and chin?	No Summer Occasionally in winter, especially around nose and mouth
8. Does your skin look tight, smooth, and ashen?	Rarely
9. Does your cleanser and moisturizer sit on top of your skin or disappear immediately into it?	Never disappears
10. How do you react to sun?	Rarely burn, good tan

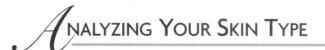

ANALYZING YOUR SKIN TYPE

We classify your skin to help you buy products that are designed for your basic skin type. These products cannot be tailored to your exact skin, however. It is like fashion designing. If you have a personal fashion designer, he or she can tailor a pattern, and change it as your body changes, to produce

COMBINATION	DRY	SENSITIVE
Sometimes: oily in spring/summer; dry in fall/winter	Rarely	Sometimes Summer problems
T-zone	T-zone Summer	T-zone Sometimes
Slightly dry-looking in appearance and feel; jawline and around eyes in fall/winter	Taut, tight, and dry in feeling and appearance with ashen, dull cast	Tight and shiny T-zone after first half-hour Sometimes in winter
Enlarged in T-zone, especially on nose, cheek, and chin	Almost invisible, fine pores	Noticeable in T-zone, fine elsewhere
T-zone problems Cheeks	Few Summer problems	Occasionally
Occasionally	Rarely Few in summer	Always Rashes and patches
Occasionally	Frequently Around eyes, forehead, mouth, lips, and chin, especially in winter	Occasionally Around eyes and nose
Sometimes Winter	Frequently, on forehead, cheeks, jawline, and chin	Rarely
Sometimes disappears	Always disappears immediately	Sometimes disappears
Slow burn, especially in summer	Burn easily without moisture protection	Burn easily without moisture protection

clothes that fit your body exactly. However, if you go to a department store, no matter how upscale it is, you must choose an item from "the rack." It could be altered to fit you, but those altered measurements are made only in a few places. In cosmetics, there are no after-purchase refinements or tailoring. You take the product from "the rack" and use it as recommended by the beauty adviser, based on the skin-type information you have provided.

In recent times, the cosmetics and beauty industry has done an excellent and thoughtful job of researching skin types. The products they offer cover

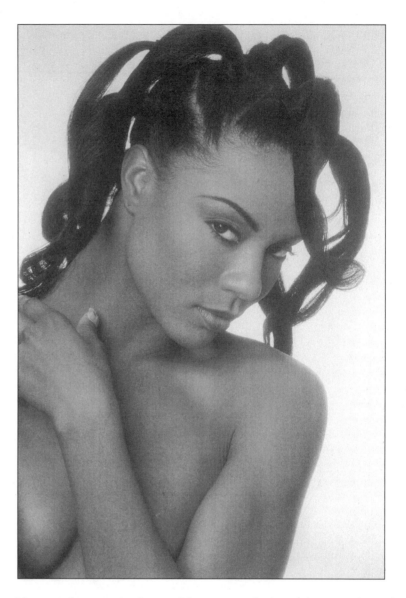

a wide enough range both to address your skin's needs properly and to enhance it while maintaining your skin's health. Answering the questions on the skin-type analysis chart can help you determine your actual skin type. Based on which column most of your answers fall into, you will know your basic skin type. You can then analyze your skin type closely enough so you will know which products to select for your skin.

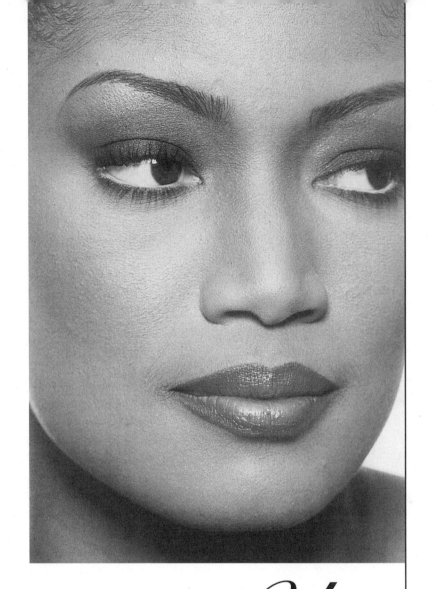

*Y*OUR
SKINCARE
REGIMEN

6

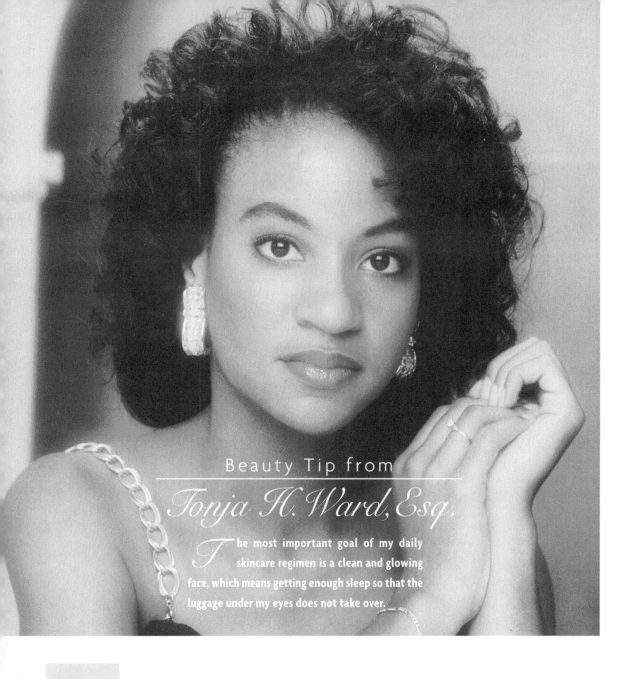

Beauty Tip from

Tonja H. Ward, Esq.

The most important goal of my daily skincare regimen is a clean and glowing face, which means getting enough sleep so that the luggage under my eyes does not take over.

Tonja H. Ward, Esq., is the wife of Charlie Ward (starting point guard for the NBA's New York Knicks) and executive vice president of Hooplife.com, the basketball Internet site that provides an inside look at the game through a daily stream of news, information, and profiles.

Now that you have determined your skin type, you can think in terms of proper facial care. When I mention "facial care," be aware that you can only address the epidermis. There are no products that penetrate deeper. Remember: proper external care and proper nutrition are two keys to healthy, beautiful skin. If you add the third key—stress reduction—your skin will be healthy and beautiful and it will also have fewer lines. And your life expectancy will be extended.

Why It Is Important to Clean Your Skin

As you know, everybody—including you—was introduced to that "bar of soap" (homemade or commercial) for "getting the dirt out." Well, we did get the dirt out and cleaned the hair, face, neck, body, and feet with the same bar of soap. The skin would feel taut and appear tight and ashen on dark skin tones and leave a reddish glow on light complexions. Most soap bars are highly alkaline, and usually the skin would become dry, irritated, patchy, blotchy, and discolored.

The hair pomades would take care of the dull hair and dry scalp. Petroleum jelly was the facial "de-asher"; and from the neck down, it was the all-purpose "ash-killer." Dirt, soot, and environmental impurities would stick to the skin and clog pores, creating excessive oiliness that would often lead to acne. The skin would take on a beautiful healthy sheen, however, which did more harm than good. Some women still use petroleum jelly products for moisture. Nevertheless, the coating properties of petroleum jelly cannot and will not moisturize the skin.

If you do not clean your skin efficiently, you can clog pores and prevent the removal of greasy dead cells while leaving a residue on your skin's surface. Your first step toward healthy skincare and maintenance is cleansing your skin properly. Clean skin imparts a soft, smooth, comfortable glow and really feels good.

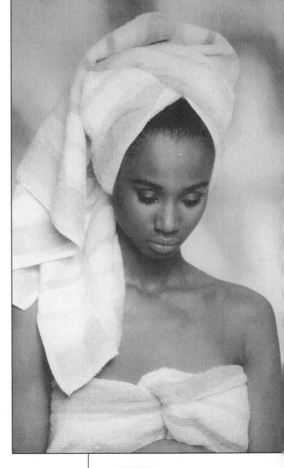

So let's start now with a proper skincare program. There are three basic steps to any quality skin regimen: cleanse, tone, moisturize. These are followed by a maintenance step, a special beauty procedure.

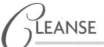LEANSE

Select a cleanser that meets the needs of your type skin, then relax your face, massaging it as described in chapter 3. See the following illustration. The cleanser will help remove the outer-cell layer and the impurities embedded in your pores. (Clogged pores are a major cause of skin eruptions and blackheads.) The cleanser should clean deep but gently.

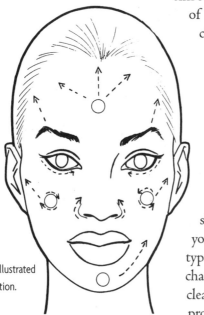

Step 1
Cleanse, following illustrated direction of application.

When choosing a cleanser for use during the summer, women with oily and combination skin should think in terms of lightweight or light-textured products such as water-soluble lotions and gels. These clean gently and have less detergent, and less of a drying effect on the skin. In the winter, women with dry skin might look to creams and rich emollients.

Try more than one of these products for your skin type, because each will be a little different. When you find the cleanser you like best, stay with it until you type your skin again, when there might be a need for a change, or if your skin reacts to the product. Facial cleansers are pH balanced and will not strip nature's protective acid mantle on your facial surface. Be aware, however, that some facial cleansers have exfoliation properties that include abrasive, mild particles that clean deep and slough away dead cells.

Remember though that your skin may not be reacting to the cleanser. First look at your diet, drinking habits, menstrual period, oral contraception use, medications, or possible pregnancy. If these are all eliminated as the cause, look to stress. When it, too, is determined not to be the cause, look at the products you are using. But generally, if properly chosen, your cleanser will not be the cause. Skin cleansers are usually well researched and tested.

ONE

Products used for toning the skin are called astringents, skin fresheners, refining lotions, or clarifying lotions. A toner rinses off any cleanser or soap film on the face. But in our regimen it does even more than that. Its other purpose is to prepare your skin to receive a moisturizer. And it has yet another purpose. Do you remember that in chapter 1, I mentioned the pH factor and the belief that the skin's natural acidity helps protect it from bacterial infection? A toner restores the pH to a proper level and corrects the balance of oil and water on the skin's surface. The preferred second step, your toner (astringent, freshener, or clarifying lotion), should be not only fragrance free, but also irritant free.

A toner is particularly important for those women with oily, dry, or sensitive skin, for it will attend to their skin's balance needs. Choose a toner suited to your skin type. Then apply it as shown in the following illustration.

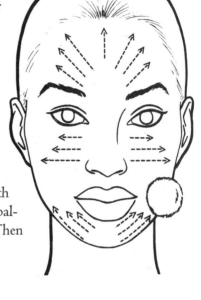

OISTURIZE

Moisturizers do different things for different skin types. However, they will do the following for all skin types: become a sealer to hold skin moisture in (emollients) and draw moisture from the air to the skin to help keep it lubricated (humectant). If your skin is dry, then your moisturizer will lubricate and protect your face with an oil-based mixture that adds necessary oil. If your skin is oily, then your moisturizer will be oil free, for your skin has all the oil it needs. The moisturizer will also be water based, fragrance free, and dermatologically tested, since oily skin has a tendency to be sensitive. Apply the moisturizer as shown in the following illustration.

As mentioned above, a moisturizer is a liquid or a cream with two critical ingredients: a humectant and emollients. A humectant attracts and absorbs moisture in and on the surface of the skin as long as possible. They

Step 2

Apply toner, following illustrated direction of application.

are either oil or nonoil substances in accordance with whether you have dry skin (oil based) or oily skin (nonoil based).

If you have combination skin, consider the time of year and the condition of your body. If it's winter and your skin is dry in places (for example, on your jaw or chin), use a moisturizer for dry skin in those areas and one for normal skin elsewhere. If it's summer and your T-zone is oily, concentrate on a moisturizer for oily skin.

All too often, women who have dry skin apply mineral oil, petroleum jelly, or cocoa butter to the eye area. This suffocates the tissue around the eyes; it cannot breathe, and it swells and gets puffy. This is exactly what you don't want. Always use a specially formulated eye oil—a lightweight, refined oil cream or gel—for this delicate area. Massage the cream or gel in, gently patting it on with your ring finger and working from the temple down to the nose. For oily skinned women, I recommend oil-free eye preparations to lubricate this area.

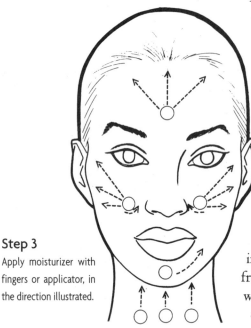

Step 3

Apply moisturizer with fingers or applicator, in the direction illustrated.

A Special Beauty Step

The special beauty step is a maintenance one. Once or twice a week, based on your skin type, you should use an exfoliating lotion, cream, or gel. These exfoliates are for deep cleansing. They reach deeper into the epidermis than can your daily cleanser.

During general cleansing each day and evening, often specific types of problem skin—for example, very dry or very oily skin—require a super cleansing. Based on the time of year and your skin type, I suggest that you indulge in weekly deep cleansing and treatment. By "deep cleansing" I mean to cleanse, tone, exfoliate, or use a mask.

If, for example, you have dry skin and it is wintertime, use a mask in spots, so as to deal exclusively with the problem area and leave the rest of your face alone. If you have oily skin and it is summertime, use an exfoliate and/or a deep-pore cleansing mask to rid your skin of dead cells and to unclog your pores.

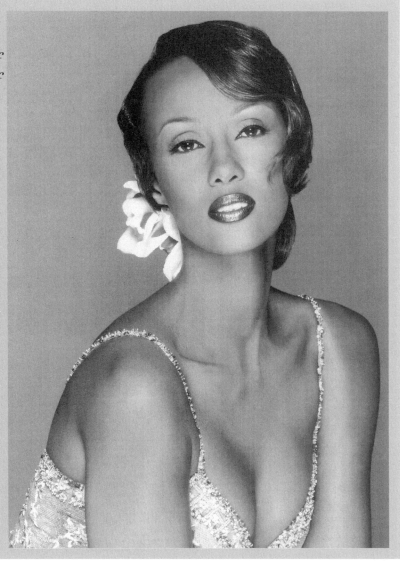

Many women have become too dependent on color systems. If you can't walk out of the house without makeup and feel great about your skin, you have problems.

—IMAN, SUPERMODEL, ACTRESS, BUSINESSWOMAN

Iman is an accomplished model and actress who has graced the covers of magazines worldwide. In her role as businesswoman, the skincare and makeup expert has created a product line specifically for women of color.

When choosing a cleanser, make sure the ingredients are not harmful or abrasive to the skin. Some general cleansers contain grains, which act as a mild exfoliate and skin stimulator. Often, the grains remove the outer layer of skin. But when the grains are chips of shells or nuts, they often have pointed, sharp edges that can scrape, split, and damage the outer layer of facial skin. Natural grains, unlike shells and nuts, are rounded and will not cut or cause such damage; they dissolve as you gently massage and scrub. My favorite scrubs are the ones with apricot and sea kelp. These facial exfoliating scrubs gently cleanse away dull skin cells for a fresh-looking complexion.

You may be thinking about one consideration I haven't yet mentioned: the eye area. This is the most delicate area, with the thinnest and fewest layers of skin. When cleansing, use the mildest nonabrasive cleansers and remember to use your fingers gently in this area and to move them from the temple toward the bridge of your nose.

Now that we have outlined the general skincare regimen, let's get specific in terms of coupling your skin type with your specific skincare regimen.

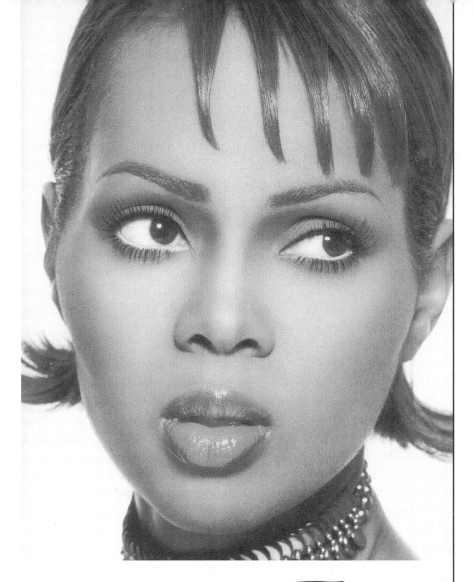

THE OILY SKIN CLASSIFICATION

7

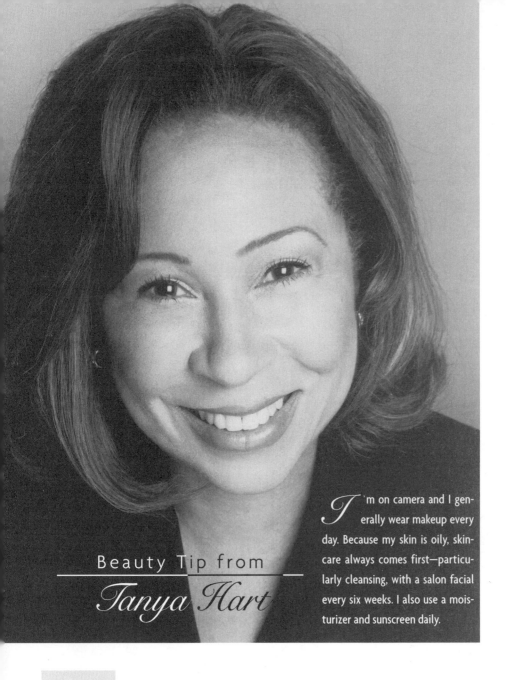

Beauty Tip from
Tanya Hart

I'm on camera and I generally wear makeup every day. Because my skin is oily, skincare always comes first—particularly cleansing, with a salon facial every six weeks. I also use a moisturizer and sunscreen daily.

Tanya Hart, as the E! Entertainment Television *Gossip Show* reporter and *National Enquirer* TV expert, has gone behind the scenes to talk about everything, giving you the juiciest information on some of today's hottest stars.

*I*f your skin is normal to oily, there is a basic regimen to help you balance and control the oil. It's important that you drink eight glasses of water a day to flush your system of internal impurities and excess oil. Your oily skin systematically produces too much oil, day and night. If the surface sebum (sebaceous oil) is not removed at least twice a day, your skin mantle collects oil, perspiration, bacteria, and impurities that will cause problems—for example, clogged pores, blackheads, and acne.

DAY CARE

PRODUCT TO USE	PRODUCT DIRECTIONS
Step 1. Cleanse Use lotion and liquid soap detergents formulated for oily skin. Nondeodorant soap bar (facial soap) also is recommended for oily skin. Use oil-free, water-based products researched for black women.	Use tepid (lukewarm) water to rinse your skin. *I do not recommend a cream cleanser on oily skin during the spring/summer months in any region.* Water-based cleansing lotions are fine if without mineral oil. (Lotion cleansers are excellent for removing stale makeup prior to deep-pore cleansing.)
	Note: Acne oily skin is a medical problem and requires the attention of a dermatologist. Ask your dermatologist about products before you purchase. Gentle facial brushes are excellent but scrubs are best to help clean clogged pores. A natural fiber puff and nonrubber cleansing brushes are recommended.
Step 2. Tone Use a fragrance-free astringent and formula for oily skin. Skin fresheners and clarifying lotions formulated for oily skin are excellent for fall/winter.	Use lavishly; apply with cotton ball or pad and wipe until clean. Avoid the eye area. Also, don't use an astringent that has resorcinol, a skin-darkening agent.
Step 3. Moisturize Use only water-based, oil-free, fragrance-free formulas for oily skin.	Light moisturizers are water-holding agents that protect, retain moisture, and shield against the environment. Place four dots of moisture lotion at the forehead, cheeks, and chin and massage into skin. No residue or tacky feeling should exist.

DAY CARE (CONT'D)

PRODUCT TO USE	PRODUCT DIRECTIONS
For lips, a mineral-oil lip moisturizer is excellent. No oil-producing glands exist on top or bottom lips, so mineral oil can seal in and protect dry tissue against the environment. Oily skin types can have dry lips during all seasons.	Apply a cocoa butter, camphor, beeswax, lanolin, or petrolatum lip moisturizer directly from the tube or pat on your lips. This formula is for lips only, and is not appropriate for the facial area ever!

Usually, oily skin is noticeably uneven in skin tone, light in the center of the face (T-zone), and slightly dark at the temples, outer cheeks, lower jawline, and chin. It is plagued with constant flare-ups and breakouts. Oily skin has visibly wide pores and a greasy, slick feeling. It can even appear dull.

EVENING CARE

PRODUCT TO USE	PRODUCT DIRECTIONS
Step 1. Cleanse	Same as for day care.
Step 2. Tone	
Step 3. Moisturize	
Special night care: use a water-based, oil-, and fragrance-free eye makeup remover.	Use product with a cotton ball or cotton eye pad to remove eye makeup. Rinse with tepid water to remove all traces.
Eye treatment: use formula for oily skin.	Sweep in gently with your ring finger from the outer corner of each eye toward the bridge of the nose.
Neck treatment: cleanse, tone, moisturize, and apply night cream or antiaging preparation.	Massage the formula into skin at the neck and throat area. See face chart, chapter 3.

A clean face is your goal. Oily skin must be washed at least once during the day and again before retiring. (The desired number of cleansings is at least three a day, reapplying fresh makeup when convenient.) Your oily skin is not a problem when you know what to do. But you must plan your time and take care to meet your skin's requirements.

PRODUCT TO USE	PRODUCT DIRECTIONS
Use a deep-pore exfoliate or scrub formulated for oily skin. Clay mask with conditioning properties is best for oily skin, especially in spring and summer, if fragrance free.	Deep-pore cleansing dislodges embedded dirt in the pores and removes the outer layer of skin-dulling dead cells. Cleansing grains are great, but avoid formulas with sharp particles, since they can scratch and scar delicate skin tissue.

Maintenance Goal

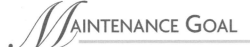

Your goal is oil control. You don't want to deplete the skin's natural oil, but you do want to kill the shine. Actually, there is an advantage to oily skin: African American women with oily skin age less and at a slower rate, owing to the oily deposits deep in the layers of the dermis. Just remember these essentials:

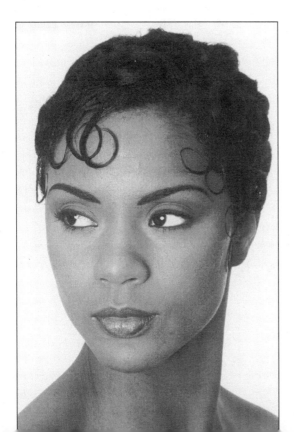

Dos and *Don'ts* for Oily Skin

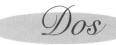

1. Do drink eight glasses of water daily.
2. Do use only water-based, oil-free, fragrance-free products.
3. Do use astringents as often as you can—day and night.
4. Do use a clay mask at least twice weekly in spring/summer, and once a week in fall/winter.
5. Do avoid fatty foods.

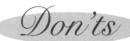

1. Don't use oil-based creams, lotions, or soaps.
2. Don't use acne-medicated cleansing pads as an astringent. You'll dry out areas around the eyes, temples, nose, and chin.
3. Don't use abrasive cleansing pads, buff puffs, or loofahs on your face frequently.
4. Don't use *pure* alcohol, witch hazel, hydrogen peroxide, or concentrated lemon juice as an astringent.

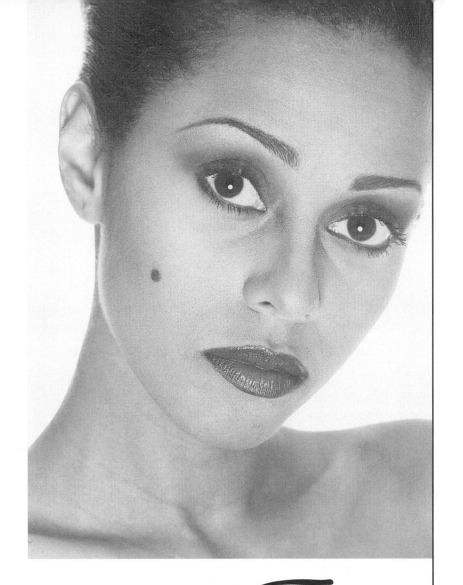

THE DRY
SKIN
CLASSIFICATION

8

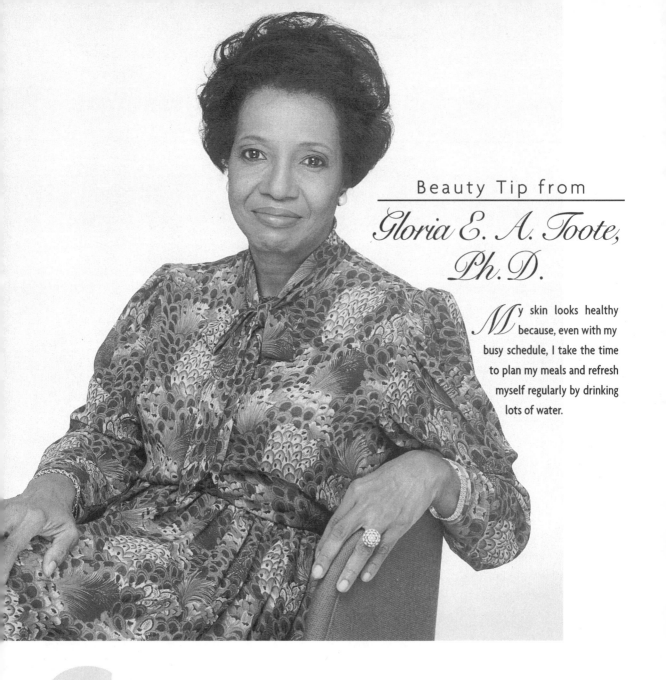

Beauty Tip from

Gloria E. A. Toote, Ph.D.

My skin looks healthy because, even with my busy schedule, I take the time to plan my meals and refresh myself regularly by drinking lots of water.

Gloria E. A. Toote, Ph.D., is an attorney, writer, building developer, and former government official. She currently officiates as CEO of Trea Estates and Enterprises, Inc., a housing development and maintenance corporation.

If your skin is normal to dry, there is a basic regimen to help you maintain a balance between moisture and oil. It's important that you try to drink eight glasses of water a day to restore the body's moisture and to flush your system of impurities. You should also know that dry skin requires serious attention.

Coating and pore-sealing oils—such as baby oil, mineral oil, and petroleum products—do not condition or relieve rough, patchy, flaking, and sometimes uncomfortably itchy skin. The ashen skin will disappear when these coating and sealing oils are applied, but they clog the pores and allow particles from the environment to stick to the skin.

DAY CARE

PRODUCT TO USE	PRODUCT DIRECTIONS
Step 1. Cleanse Select a dry-skin oil cleanser if your skin is extremely dry; a rich, creamy formula if your skin is moderately dry; and, if you are a soap-and-water person, a non-deodorant formula with rich emollients and conditioners designed for dry skin.	Tissue or rinse off. Massage gently, always moving upward and outward; see face chart in chapter 3. Rinse with tepid water until your face is absolutely clean.
Step 2. Tone Use a nonalcohol toner for extremely dry skin or a low-alcohol toner for moderately dry skin.	Apply with a cotton ball or pad and wipe until all traces of surface impurities are gone.
Step 3. Moisturize Select a rich dry-skin emollient with moisturizers and conditioners specifically for dry skin. I prefer the fragrance-free dermatologically tested formulas.	Smooth in gently from the base of your neck, massaging from the throat area upward to the hairline.
Your lips suffer in the winter. Use a mineral-oil lip preparation to trap and seal moisture on your lips. Medicated formulas relieve cracked, peeling, bleeding, and splitting.	Gently smooth in the penetrating emollient. Do not apply this formula to your face.

EVENING CARE

PRODUCT TO USE	PRODUCT DIRECTIONS
Step 1. Cleanse	Same as for day care.
Step 2. Tone	
Step 3. Moisturize	
Special night care: use a no-tear, fragrance-free, dermatologically tested makeup remover.	Use product with a cotton ball or cotton pad to remove eye makeup. Rinse with tepid water to remove all traces.
Eye treatment: use a rich, light-textured emollient.	Sweep in gently with your ring finger from the outer corner of each eye toward the bridge of the nose.
Antiaging treatment: use a night cream or antiaging cell-renewal formula for your extremely dry, line- and wrinkle-prone skin. Mature dry skin may require a special firming cream or lotion to help soften and smooth the skin and restore a healthy glow.	Massage formula into skin or neck, throat, face, ears, and at hairline.

Dry skin can look dull and gray or ashen, be sensitive, and often be painful. Its fine pores can clog and break out. The problem areas are the forehead, lower cheeks, jawline, and chin. A dry, peeling nose can have fine dirt imbedded as blackheads and whiteheads on the side and tip, invisible and unnoticeable but sensitive to the touch. Dry skin reacts to extreme cold and hot temperatures, and suffers from a lack of both internal and surface moisture (dehydration) as well as from inadequate production of surface oil

WEEKLY CARE

PRODUCT TO USE	PRODUCT DIRECTIONS
Use a moisturizing cream to slough and peel off dry skin. (If you have thick facial hair, the peel-off type is not recommended.) Avoid clay or drawing formulas because they remove too much natural oil and moisture.	Apply a thin film of moisturizer over extremely dry skin before applying a gel peel-off mask. Cream the mask with healing conditioners—e.g., aloe vera.

(sebum). Dry skin ages faster than oily or combination skin. The result can be premature wrinkles and crepey-looking lines around the eyes and mouth.

MAINTENANCE GOALS

Your goal is to replenish and maintain the balance of water and oil on your delicate skin surface. You want to rid the skin of dulling dead facial cells and impurities. You must take every preventive step to lubricate and hold moisture on your skin. Harsh winter and summer air robs your skin of its natural moisture and oil. You can retard the deepening and lining of your face with proper care and with moisture-conditioning formulas that penetrate the layers of the epidermis. Here are your essentials:

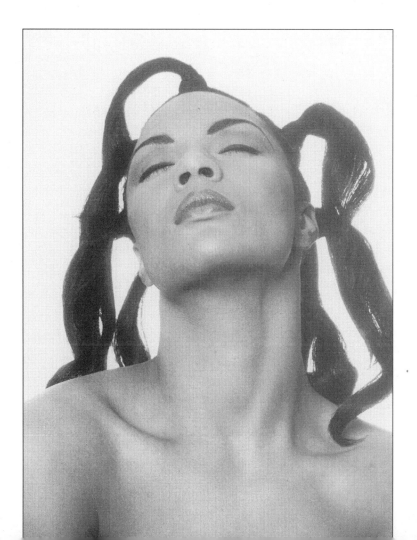

Dos and *Don'ts* for Dry Skin

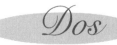

Dos

1. Do drink eight glasses of water daily.
2. Do use only oil-based, moisture-conditioning, dermatologically tested products.
3. Do use a cream mask for very dry skin.
4. Do ventilate your daytime and evening rooms. Humidifiers are an excellent way to control moisture.
5. Do use spot facial masks during summer and winter, applying them to problem areas only.

Don'ts

1. Don't use astringents formulated for oily and combination skin.
2. Don't use abrasive, exfoliating granular-based masks.
3. Don't use deodorant-type soaps on your face. From the neck down, deodorant soaps are fine.
4. Don't use petroleum jelly, cocoa butter, mineral oil, or baby oil as a facial moisturizer, especially if you are going to wear a cream or liquid-cream makeup foundation. However, cocoa butter and petroleum by-products are excellent for the lower body parts.

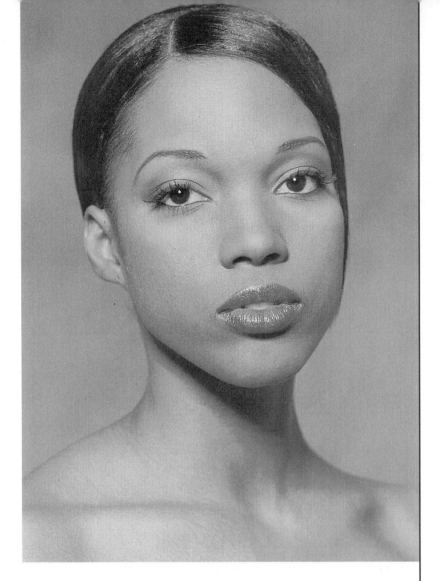

THE COMBINATION
SKIN
CLASSIFICATION

9

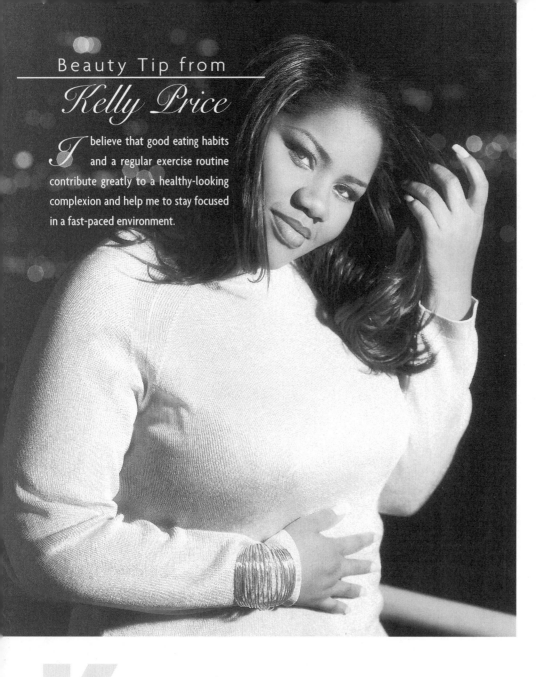

Beauty Tip from
Kelly Price

I believe that good eating habits and a regular exercise routine contribute greatly to a healthy-looking complexion and help me to stay focused in a fast-paced environment.

Kelly Price has a long list of credits, as a songwriter, background vocalist, and arranger for performers. Her debut on Island Black Music was *Soul of a Woman,* which sold over a million copies, and she received a Grammy nomination for best R & B performance by a duo or group on Whitney Houston's "Heartbreak Hotel."

Your skin may be oily, dry, or sensitive in different areas, and it requires special attention in both summer and winter. There is a basic regimen you should follow to maintain a balance between moisture and oil. It's important that you drink eight glasses of water a day to flush your system of internal impurities and to restore the balance of water and oil on the surface of the skin.

DAY CARE

PRODUCT TO USE	PRODUCT DIRECTIONS
Step 1. Cleanse Use a liquid soap with mild detergent and facial shampoo properties. There are water-based lotions and nondrying facial cleansing soap bars designed for normal to combination skin.	Splash on water and rinse thoroughly with tepid water. Use the face chart in chapter 3 for proper movement directions as you massage.
Step 2. Tone Use an astringent for oily zones in summer. Use a skin freshener for normal to dry zones in winter.	Dampen a cotton ball or pad and wipe until ball or pad is absolutely clean.
Step 3. Moisturize Use a lotion or lightweight soufflé-type (has a whipped cream texture, or "foamy") moisturizer.	For summer oiliness, apply oil-free moisturizer all over, from neck to forehead. For winter dryness, apply soufflé-type moisturizer cream. Apply moisturizer with fingers or applicator in the direction illustrated on page 54.
For lips, in winter use a moisturizer.	Apply directly from the tube or pat on.

When in balance, a combination skin can actually be normal. But seasonal conditions can affect combination skin to the point where it may be normal during one season and dry or oily during another. Additionally, stress, a dramatic weight loss or gain, dietary food changes, an irregular menstrual cycle, and aging can disturb the natural balance of acidity, moisture, oil, and dryness.

Skin eruptions, breakouts, and patchy rashes can sometimes occur on your forehead, cheeks, and chin. Your pores are fine around the hairline, temples, chin, and jawline but visible in the T-zone. Your skin can be part oily

EVENING CARE	
PRODUCT TO USE	**PRODUCT DIRECTIONS**
Step 1. Cleanse	Same as for day care.
Step 2. Tone	
Step 3. Moisturize	
Special night care: use eye makeup remover for combination-type skin.	Use product with a cotton ball or cotton pad to remove eye makeup. Rinse with tepid water to remove all traces.
Eye treatment: use formulas appropriate for dry and oily eye zones.	Using the ring finger, gently apply eye preparation over and under the eye.

and part dry at the same time, so you must select appropriate treatment products for different areas of your face and times of year.

WEEKLY CARE	
PRODUCT TO USE	**PRODUCT DIRECTIONS**
Antiaging treatment: use cell-renewal firming lotions or creams and night creams designed for dry and oily skin.	A few drops of this firming formula is applied to the problem aging areas.
Problem areas: use a clay mask for oily areas. A creamy mask with soft grains helps draw out toxins and heals, firms, and alleviates whiteheads and blackheads.	Spot-mask the oily areas twice a month in the summer and once a month in the winter for six to ten minutes. Avoid applying clay mask to dry areas of face.

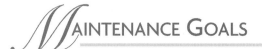

MAINTENANCE GOALS

Your goals are to treat, care for, and maintain your normal to combination skin. Your emphasis in summer should be on the oily zones and in winter on healing and conditioning the dry areas. Weekly deep-pore cleansing is important. Just be sure to remember these essentials:

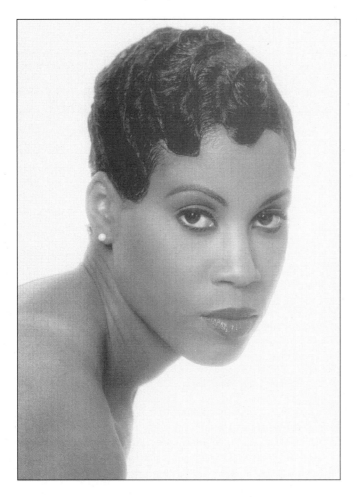

Dos and *Don'ts* for Combination Skin

Dos

⚬ ⚬ ⚬ ⚬ ⚬ ⚬ ⚬ ⚬ ⚬ ⚬ ⚬ ⚬ ⚬ ⚬ ⚬ ⚬ ⚬ ⚬

1. Do drink eight glasses of water daily.

2. Do use during the summer season oil-free products that are light in texture.

3. Do choose skin fresheners and toners formulated for normal and combination skin, based on the season.

4. Do use products formulated and tested for normal and combination skin.

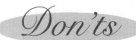

1. Don't use the same product year-round. Your skin type changes dramatically. Observe your skin and note the oily and dry areas.

2. Don't use abrasive cosmetic tools over the entire face, especially in the winter months.

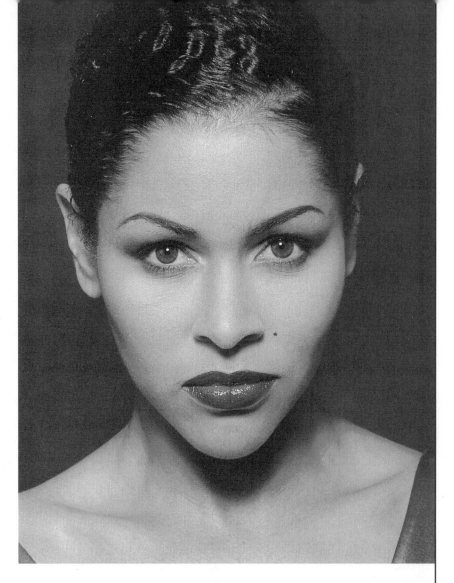

THE SENSITIVE SKIN CLASSIFICATION

10

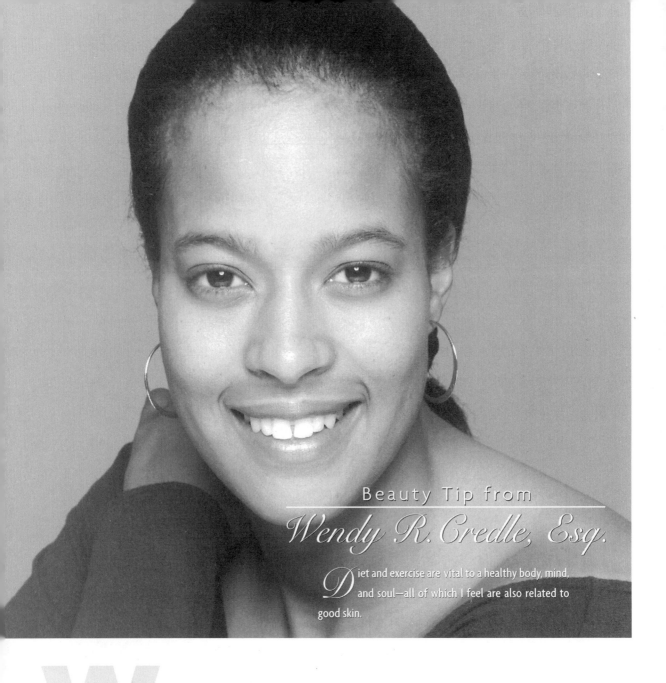

Beauty Tip from

Wendy R. Credle, Esq.

*D*iet and exercise are vital to a healthy body, mind, and soul—all of which I feel are also related to good skin.

Wendy R. Credle, Esq. is counsel at the entertainment firm of Rudolph & Beer, LLP, where she specializes in music and represents many distinguished artists, producers, writers, and executives.

If your skin is sensitive, there is a basic regimen that will calm, balance, and alleviate discomfort. It's important that you drink eight glasses of water daily to rid your body of external impurities. Use fragrance-, irritant-, and oil-free products that are hypoallergenic or have been dermatologically tested.

Your skin type has less tolerance of chemical substances and reacts to poor dietary habits, stress, hormonal changes, allergies, trauma, and impurities in the environment, exfoliating creams and lotions, and plastic surgery.

DAY CARE

PRODUCT TO USE	PRODUCT DIRECTIONS
Step 1. Cleanse In summer, use a lotion, liquid soap, or facial soap bar. In winter, use a liquid cream or cream formula that is fragrance- and oil-free. Use products tested for black sensitive skin.	Massage liquid facial soap or lotion gently with your fingertips, using the face chart in chapter 3. Rinse thoroughly. Tissue off or rinse off water-soluble creams.
Note: Do not squeeze acne pimples, or dark scarring may occur. Do not use harsh cleansers or scrubs. Do not aggravate overactive oil glands or eruptions. Preparations are on the market to correct young people's and adult acne. See a dermatologist.	
Step 2. Tone Use a skin freshener designed for black sensitive skin, with low or no alcohol or resorcinol. Skin fresheners fight bacteria, balance the oil and moisture levels on your skin, and refine the pores.	Wipe the entire face, avoiding eye zones, until a cotton pad or ball is absolutely clean.
Step 3. Moisturize Use fragrance-free and oil-free lotions, or light, creamy soufflé-type moisturizers, that are formulated for black sensitive skin. Fragrance- and oil-free moisturizers are water-holding agents to protect, condition, and smooth surface tissue.	In summer, your skin does not need a coating or sealing of moisturizer. In winter, apply a light film of cream.

EVENING CARE	
PRODUCT TO USE	**PRODUCT DIRECTIONS**
Step 1. Cleanse	Same as for day care.
Step 2. Tone	
Step 3. Moisturize	
Special night care: use a no-tear, fragrance-free, hypoallergenic, dermatologically tested eye makeup remover.	Use product with a cotton ball or cotton pad to remove eye makeup. Rinse with tepid water to remove all traces.
Eye treatment: use a cream designed for dry and sensitive skin.	Sweep in from the outer corner of each eye, toward the bridge of the nose, gently applying the cream with your ring finger.
Antiaging treatment: use a cell-renewal preparation for sensitive skin.	Massage formula into skin on neck, throat, face, and at hairline.

It tends to be drier in certain areas and may have frequent skin eruptions. Your skin may bruise easily, resulting in dark spots. Cosmetics companies have made excellent efforts to meet the needs of your sensitive skin, with products that are dermatologically tested to heal, soothe, and relieve your skin conditions and to improve your skin texture.

I recommend that you consult a dermatologist for treating extreme or severe sensitive skin conditions. Also, have a cosmetologist, aesthetician, or beauty adviser do a patch test before you purchase a new product; you might even take a sample of that product to your dermatologist.

WEEKLY CARE	
PRODUCT TO USE	**PRODUCT DIRECTIONS**
Problem areas: use a clay or drawing-formula mask to lift blackheads and draw out toxins and other impurities. Use peel-off or moisture-conditioning masks to clean deep, lifting away accumulated dead cells.	In summer, spot-mask problem oily areas only. (Not recommended for dry areas.) In winter, spot-mask on dry skin zones only.

MAINTENANCE GOAL

Your goal is to be as gentle as possible with your skin. Attend to breakouts or acne eruptions immediately. Your hands and fingertips carry microorganisms that breed on dirt, stale makeup, and polluted oil, so keep hands and fingers off your face.

You must select a treatment system from one cosmetics company. Do not mix treatment products. (For example, don't combine cleanser from X, toner from Y, and moisturizer from Z.) Fragrance- and oil-free, water-based products that have been tested by dermatologists are recommended.

Now you know your skin type and have a regimen for daily care. You should, however, take into account the season—spring/summer or fall/winter—when you answer the skin-typing questionnaire. And don't forget to ask yourself if there are any special changes going on: Are you dieting? Do you have your period? Been doing a "lot of partying"? I am sure you know this already, for I mentioned it early on, but it's worth repeating. Since the germinating layer of your skin is fed through your blood system, what you eat and what gets into your blood system have a noticeable effect on your face. Here, then, are your essential dos and don'ts.

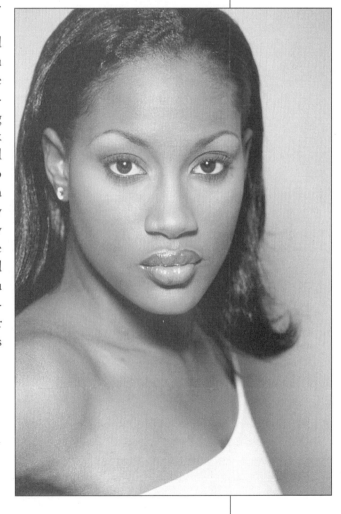

Dos and *Don'ts* for Sensitive Skin

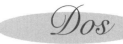

Dos

1. Do drink eight glasses of water daily.
2. Do use acne-cleansing pads without resorcinol, which when used on black skin acts as a darkening agent.
3. Do stay calm and learn to relax to help chase skin problems away.
4. Do develop better dietary habits. What you put in your body affects your skin.
5. Do use special astringent or skin fresheners formulated for sensitive skin.
6. Do keep your face's dry zones in check.

Don'ts

1. Don't use astringents designed for oily skin on dry zones of your face.
2. Don't eat a lot of dairy products, salty and oily foods, or sugar-filled products, including chocolate.

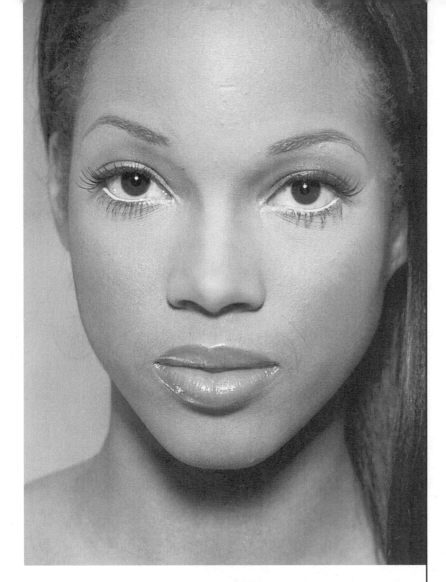

COLORING YOUR
SKIN

11

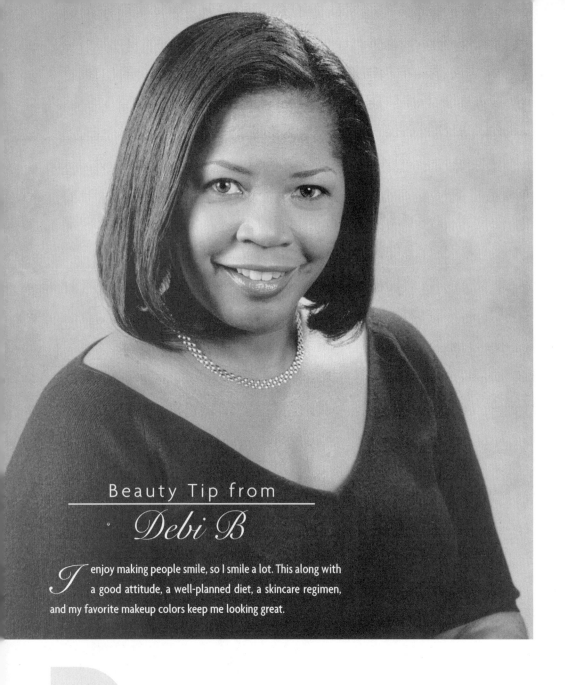

Debi B

I enjoy making people smile, so I smile a lot. This along with a good attitude, a well-planned diet, a skincare regimen, and my favorite makeup colors keep me looking great.

Deborah Bolling Jackson ("Debi B") cohosts *The Sunday Classics* every Sunday morning on 107.5 WBLS Radio opposite her legendary husband, Hal Jackson. She is also the producer of the Hal Jackson's Talented Teens International Competition.

The most notable factors determining your best makeup colors are your facial skin color, your hair color, and your eye color. Black women today can change their hair color and can appear to have changed their eye color by wearing tinted contact lenses; to some degree, they can even lighten their skin color with bleaching agents or darken it through tanning. But even if you do all this, you will still have three colors to consider: your hair, eye, and skin colors.

Of these three colors, your skin color is the most important classification. There are at least sixteen million African American women in the United States, and there are thirty-nine recognized colors of black skin. (White skin has approximately eight to ten skin colors.) So you can readily understand why you need to spend more time understanding your skin color and in choosing the right products to enhance it. Using makeup colors designed for white skin will probably result in inappropriate choices. This is because a white woman can apply a much wider range of colors to her face with less negative effect, since she's probably starting with a neutral skin color.

*Y*OUR FACIAL SKIN COLOR

Let's start at the beginning. Skin color is determined by three factors: carotene, melanin, and hemoglobin. Carotene gives a yellowish tinge to the skin, while melanin lends a brown color, and hemoglobin contributes a reddish hue to the skin. The more melanin, the darker the surface skin tone; carotene, on the other hand, provides contrast with a yellow undertone. The tone and undertone to your skin are based on the amount of carotene and melanin in the epidermis. For example, there are Africans from the Sudan who are so dark that they appear to have a bluish aura to their skin. This is directly related to the amount of epidermal melanin and hemoglobin.

All makeup is created to complement the undertone as well as the surface tone of your face. You may have forgotten the basic color chart, but now you need to know that, in terms of primary colors, brown is really a red. There is a range of colors, or shades, that you should use in your makeup, based on the amount and quality of color in your skin. Although the range of possible colors is wide, it is not limitless. Some colors do not go well with other

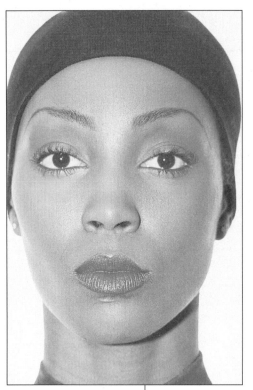

colors. And the more facial colors you have to work with, the more limited are your makeup options. The colors you put on your face should go well with the colors of your hair, eyes, and skin and should appeal to your sense of self as well as be appropriate for the occasion.

Color Coding

Cosmetics manufacturers today often classify white skin color by seasons of the year. Those colors that lie within a certain range are called winter colors or fall colors; those that lie within the other range are called summer or spring colors. This may make fashion sense to some, but black skin requires an entirely different classification system.

Among women of color are those who are fair-skinned, with blonde or ash blond to light-brown hair. Then there are women who have medium-light to dark-brown hair. There are also women with dark-brown to black hair. And finally, there are women with blue-black hair. For example, Trinidadians often have "coal black" hair, which has a bluish cast.

As you can see, I am relating hair color to skin color. Skin color bears a relationship to your natural hair color; therefore, your natural skin color is the key to determining your best fashion and cosmetics colors.

The other feature you need to remember in color coding is your eyes. For blacks, the eye range is from green to hazel, blue to hazel, hazel to light brown, dark brown, and very dark brown. Also, there is a special category for the eye color that people from the Caribbean and sometimes Africa have: hazel eyes with a bluish outer rim.

The Fornay Color Chart is far more relevant than the seasons for black women, and using it requires far greater care. Makeup for blacks calls for a more delicate balance of colors and shades. Once you know your colors, you can decide which ones look best on

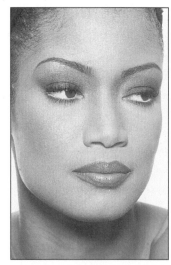

you. The right color choices will help make you feel the way you wish to feel and look the way you wish to look.

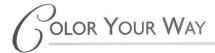

COLOR YOUR WAY

Way back when, you probably once said, "I don't know what colors to wear." Over the years you decided—or someone else decided for you—which colors were best on your face and what colors were best in your wardrobe. Well, maybe you were right and maybe you were wrong.

Be daring enough to go on this color journey with me and see if the colors you chose are indeed your best colors and whether they really please you. Remember: no matter how much a color "may be for you," if you are unhappy with it then it isn't really for you. Color not only makes you look a certain way, but it also makes you feel a certain way as well. And how you feel will affect how you look.

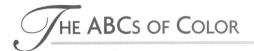

THE ABCs OF COLOR

Don't let the myriad eye shadows, blushers, lipsticks, and nail polishes throw you. There are hundreds of hues but only three basic colors: red, yellow, and blue. This is as important to remember as the fact that black skin generally has one of the following three undertones: yellow, brown, or red-blue, with all their gradations.

You also need to remember that a color will draw from itself. For example, yellow will draw from orange, making the orange look more red. Why does this occur? Since orange is a combination of yellow and red, the yellows are pulled to each other (the yellow in your skin's undertone and the yellow in the color), in a sense leaving the red to stand alone, complementing the yellow.

So, if you have a sallow complexion or a yellow, yellow-red, yellow-beige, or even olive undertone, then red is an inviting color. On the other hand, if you have more of a ruddy complexion, with a more red than yellow undertone, the red draws from the orange, leaving a yellow look. In the same way, if you use green eye shadow and have blue eyes, your eye color drains the blue from the green, leaving a yellow look.

Even though this principle may seem easy, it can get complicated. My color chart in the middle of the book takes into account the colors of your hair, skin, and eyes.

There are two factors, however, that the color chart does not address. For these, only you or your situation can determine the best colors. First, some colors make you *feel* warm, vibrant, and alive, while others make you *feel* cool, "laid-back," and somber. There are sufficient colors in each skin, hair, and eye category to permit you to choose the right color for the mood you want.

Second, certain colors may be more appropriate than others for a particular time of day, occasion, and fashion. You can make the correct choices from your category, since each has enough colors from which to select.

Forget the Color Seasons

You may be surprised that I have not presented colors in terms of seasons of the year. This is because I believe a black woman doesn't need a certain season to wear a given color. She can make herself feel like any season she wants. There is no reason why you can't wear "summer" colors in the winter or "spring" colors in the fall. In fact, you will find any color in nature during any season, someplace in the world. So far, I have noted the three guides you have in determining what colors to put on your face: your skin tone, your eye color, and your hair color. Those three do not clash with one another. One way or another, they are in harmony, and that is the key. The color you put on your face must harmonize with each feature individually and all three collectively. When this occurs, the invisible fourth guide—the "plus"—comes into play: how you feel and wish to feel.

Don't get caught by the notion that colors should be more subdued in the winter and brighter in the summer. Camouflage may help animals protect themselves from predators by allowing them to blend into their surroundings. But you are a proud, lovely black woman who wishes to make a harmonious statement, so make the statement. My color chart helps you make yourself up without either disappearing into the background or clashing with it. It allows you to be yourself.

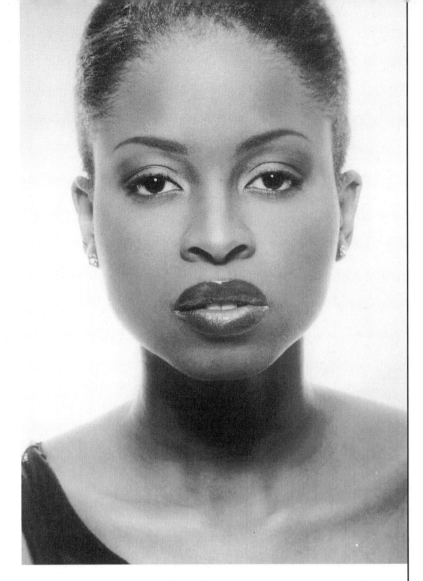

$\mathcal{F}$OUNDATIONS
FOR YOUR
SKIN TYPE

12

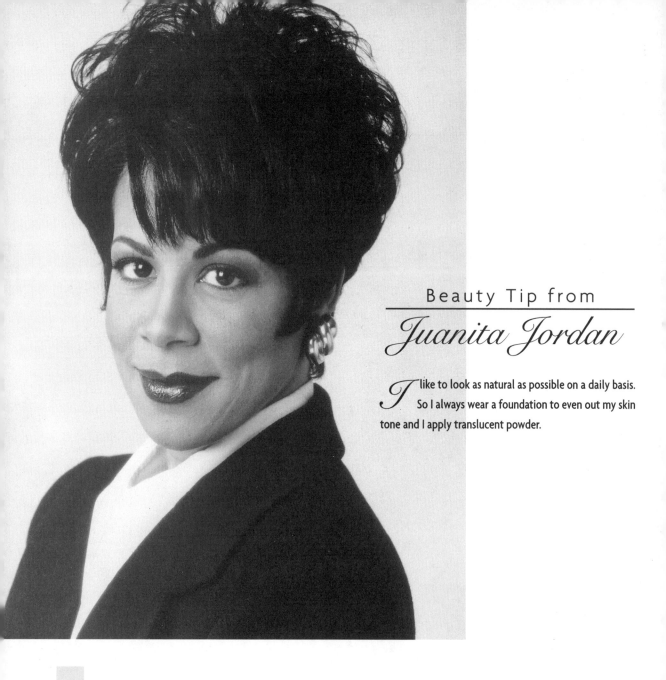

Beauty Tip from
Juanita Jordan

I like to look as natural as possible on a daily basis. So I always wear a foundation to even out my skin tone and I apply translucent powder.

Juanita Jordan, wife of basketball legend Michael Jordan, is cofounder of The Michael and Juanita Jordan (M & J) Endowment Fund, a private family fund that supports a variety of community and educational institutions and is an active supporter of Chicago's major cultural institutions.

The Fornay

COLOR CHART

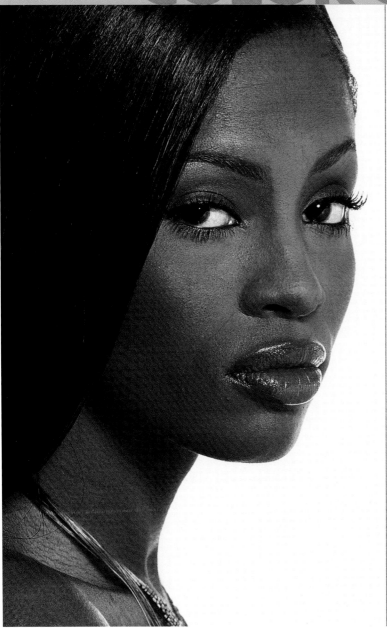

The Fornay Color Chart is a guide to selecting your best cosmetic and fashion colors. I have put it together just for you to represent the diverse hues of the African American woman's skin, eye, and hair color.

Your COLOR CHART

MATCHING FASHION COLORS WITH YOUR SKIN COLOR

Dark Skin

Dark complexions with grayed and red undertones look best with primary hues of red, mauve, and magenta.

Suggested colors:

- ■ Red Violet/Fuschia
- ■ Deep Black
- ■ Burgundy
- ■ Green
- ■ Lavender
- ■ Blue/Blue Violet
- ■ Tan
- ■ Hunter Green

Complimentary accent colors are: Yellow, Orange, Deep Gold, Black, and Chartreuse.

Medium Skin

Medium-brown and dark complexions usually look best in shades that have a bit of red added to them. In general, they are flattered by colors with blue undertones, rather than yellow.

Suggested colors:

- ■ Pink
- ■ Lavender
- ■ Royal Blue
- ■ Warm Gray
- ■ Black
- ■ Blue-Green
- ■ Peach
- ■ Blue Violet
- ■ Gray

Complimentary accent colors are: Brilliant Red, Teal, and Orange Tonal Blacks with neutral characteristics such as Gray or Black.

Light Skin

Fair, light skin with yellow or olive coloring will usually look best in shades that have an earthy yellow cast.

Suggested colors:

- ■ Coral
- ■ Vivid Orange Red
- ■ Yellow Green
- ■ Pastel Cream
- ■ Eggshell Yellow

Complimentary accent colors are: Violet, Brown, Terra Cotta, Amber, and Greenish Blue.

Best Cosmetic & Fashion Colors to Select for Your Skin, Hair, Eyes, and Total Look

MATCHING COSMETIC COLORS WITH YOUR EYE COLOR

The color of your eyes and their hues are illuminated if you wear a shade that matches or is slightly darker than your eye coloring. If you have light brown, hazel, blue-green, or green eyes, experiment with wearing a softer shade of eye color near the bridge of the nose and a more intense shade farther away to contour the eyes.

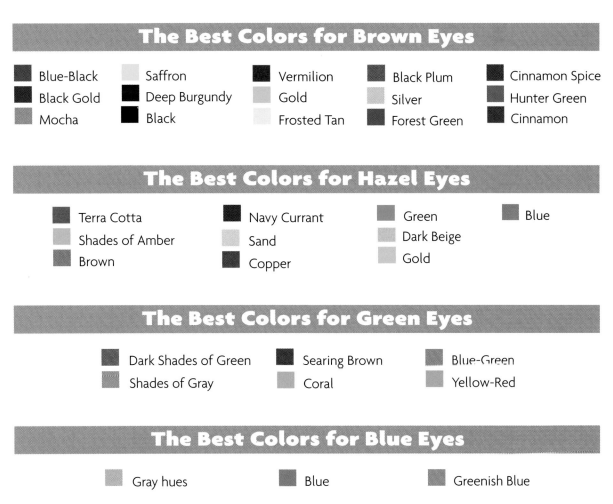

The Best Colors for Brown Eyes

- Blue-Black
- Black Gold
- Mocha
- Saffron
- Deep Burgundy
- Black
- Vermilion
- Gold
- Frosted Tan
- Black Plum
- Silver
- Forest Green
- Cinnamon Spice
- Hunter Green
- Cinnamon

The Best Colors for Hazel Eyes

- Terra Cotta
- Shades of Amber
- Brown
- Navy Currant
- Sand
- Copper
- Green
- Dark Beige
- Gold
- Blue

The Best Colors for Green Eyes

- Dark Shades of Green
- Shades of Gray
- Searing Brown
- Coral
- Blue-Green
- Yellow-Red

The Best Colors for Blue Eyes

- Gray hues
- Blue
- Greenish Blue

Best Cosmetic & Fashion Colors to Select for Your Skin, Hair, Eyes, and Total Look

MATCHING LIPSTICK AND BLUSH TO YOUR SKIN COLOR

When choosing your lipstick and blusher, always keep them in the same color family so that they don't clash. For instance, a red lipstick will call for a red-toned blusher; brown tones or earth tones coordinate well with spice tones. To set a mood or make a statement, consider the intensity of the tones or colors you choose. Reds are strong and suggest assertiveness; oranges are more sporty or casual; brown tones work well when you want to be more professionally polished; and pinks offer just a suggestion of color for a more natural look. Always make sure your lipstick and blush colors accent your wardrobe and complement your eyeshadow as well.

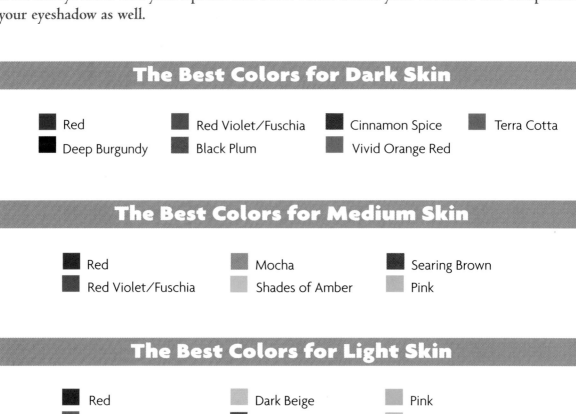

The Best Colors for Dark Skin

- Red
- Deep Burgundy
- Red Violet/Fuschia
- Black Plum
- Cinnamon Spice
- Vivid Orange Red
- Terra Cotta

The Best Colors for Medium Skin

- Red
- Red Violet/Fuschia
- Mocha
- Shades of Amber
- Searing Brown
- Pink

The Best Colors for Light Skin

- Red
- Coral
- Dark Beige
- Copper
- Pink
- Shades of Amber

Many people think that foundation is just a concealer. But really it's used to impart a hint of color to your skin. Foundation is sometimes referred to as "base," "base color," or "makeup base." When I talk to African American women about foundation, I stress that foundation has several uses.

USES FOR FOUNDATION

1. Protects against bacteria and impurities.

2. Evens out the skin tones—that is, a light T-zone or dark patchy areas.

3. Improves skin texture for a flawless, smooth finish; blushers and other makeup glide on easier and cling better when the skin is veiled with a foundation.

4. Kills or decreases sallow skin (a greenish-yellowish or ashy cast), which happens with certain skin pigment types.

5. Creates a natural-looking healthy skin glow.

HOW TO CHOOSE YOUR FOUNDATION

African American women should choose a foundation that perfectly matches their skin tone. To be able to choose properly, first there are some "don'ts" you should avoid.

Test the center of your face, cheeks, and jawline to determine a perfect foundation match.

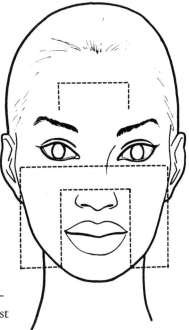

Don'ts

1. Don't try to change your skin tone with foundation. Black models, actresses, entertainers, and opera stars have to change their skin tone to create a stage effect. However, most women appear in natural light or artificial light. It is important to choose a foundation that coordinates and harmonizes with your skin tone.

2. Don't buy a foundation without testing several colors in your skin-tone range. Test them in natural and artificial light.

3. Don't buy one foundation and expect it to impart the right color for four seasons of the year.

4. Don't wear your friends' foundations. If a friend is in your color range, she might have yellow-olive undertones whereas you might have yellow-red. The foundation will therefore be different.

5. Don't rush your purchase. You can't rush into a store on the tail end of your lunch hour and quickly choose the foundation, especially if it's your first time or you have developed new color problems. You must take the time and have the patience to test your foundation, but first check your skin for changes and buy foundation accordingly.

Now that those don'ts are out of the way, here's what you should do. First, because your skin is dark, it is important that you test a foundation

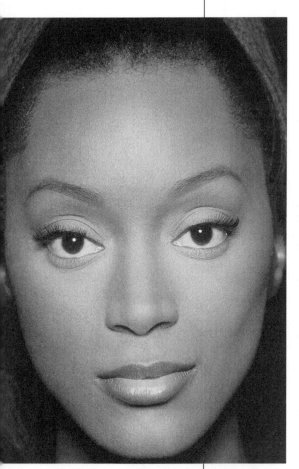

based on the season when it is to be worn. As your skin gets darker or lighter, it can take on a golden-red, reddish-brown, or brownish-blue undertone based on the amount of sun or wind it is exposed to. Don't look for an exact match; you are not involved in true skin-tone matching. For example, in the summer I suggest a summer foundation that cools down the yellow, red, and blue undertones.

A black woman's true skin tone can be tested for accuracy during the latter part of the fall and in the winter months. The situation is different, however, for light, medium, and dark skin tones, for they turn sallow, olive-brown, or deepish yellow-gray or brown. I suggest a winter foundation that imparts golden-beige, copper-brown, and rich red-brown radiance to African skin tones.

Second, you should be aware that there are now fifteen cosmetics companies marketing skin-bleaching agents to black women. These products permit you to even out your skin tone or fade out blotches and superficial spots. The bleaching product blends the shades of the spot and the surrounding skin. These creams also lighten the outer layer, giving an appearance of lighter skin. You should remember something when you use these bleaching creams. Your skin takes on a more yellowish undertone, since you have bleached out the dark part of the brown pigment in the melanin. This slight difference means you must rematch your foundation.

Third, you should know the effects of your medications. Birth control pills will often darken large parts of your face. Medicine for high blood pressure will sometimes cause the skin to take on a deeper, reddish-brown or gray-brown undertone. A liver condition, excessive alcohol consumption, and drug abuse will darken a large section of your face. When such conditions take place, you must revise your foundation. You may have to change the shade until your skin color returns to normal.

Last, make an appointment with a makeup artist or beauty adviser in a retail store or salon. Have the individual do a full-scale makeup application. Refer to our discussion of what you should expect from your makeup, and see the foundation chart on page 92 and color chart in the middle of the book.

Your skin's undertone, as discussed earlier, is the aura or glow of your true skin tone. It can be flushed out by standing in a room or in front of a white wall, with white background, and in natural light. Wrap your hair with your whitest scarf or drape your neck and shoulders with a white sheet. Allow the ultraviolet light to bounce off your face until you can actually see a green (olive), yellow, reddish-yellow, reddish-brown, or blue aura.

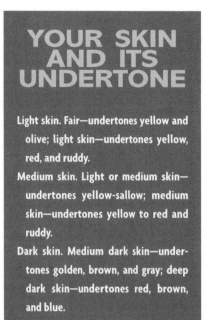

YOUR SKIN AND ITS UNDERTONE

Light skin. Fair—undertones yellow and olive; light skin—undertones yellow, red, and ruddy.

Medium skin. Light or medium skin—undertones yellow-sallow; medium skin—undertones yellow to red and ruddy.

Dark skin. Medium dark skin—undertones golden, brown, and gray; deep dark skin—undertones red, brown, and blue.

COSMETICS TERMINOLOGY

There are the generic color categories the cosmetics companies use to describe the skin of African American women. For instance, beige becomes Golden Beige by Company X. Amber becomes Amber Gold by Company Y, and cocoa becomes Cocoa Beige by Company Z. When companies refer to colors in the light-skin category, the generic words are *alabaster, beige, amber, tawny, café au lait.* The cosmetics trade uses the following when describing medium skin: *cinnamon, copper, bronze, light brown.* They refer to the colors of dark skin as *teak, cocoa, dark brown, mahogany.* There are many, many more terms, but these are examples of how the cosmetics industry classifies skin tones and how it tries to give exciting and flattering names to the colors it wants you to buy.

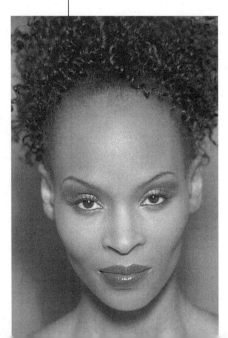

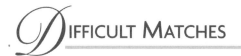

DIFFICULT MATCHES

For all their research, there is a skin tone that cosmetics companies find difficult to match. It is the tone in the medium range that has yellow or sallow, ruddy undertones. With some searching and patience, however, even this skin tone can be matched to a color foundation.

I have no respect for retail beauty advisers or makeup artists who suggest that a customer mix shades to achieve a match. These advisers don't have the shade themselves, are not knowledgeable, or only want to take your money. If the customer is foolish enough, she will have spent as much as seventy dollars for one shade of foundation to match her skin. Even the wealthy would balk at this price, particularly when the foundation probably costs about forty dollars. With so many foundations being produced for black skin, blending is rarely needed.

Companies and general manufacturers who market beauty products for blacks have researched and developed foundations in literally hundreds of

TYPES OF FOUNDATION

SKIN TYPE	FORMULA	COVERAGE	TEXTURE
Oily (use oil-free base)	Liquid/summer	Light	Matte
	Cream/winter	Medium/total	Semimatte
	Cream to powder/ summer	Medium	Matte
Dry (use oil-based makeup)	Pancake cream	Total	Dewy
	Soufflé cream	Medium/total	Dewy
	Stick/tube	Total	Dewy
	Liquid	Sheer/medium	Semimatte
Combination (use water-based makeup)	Liquid	Sheer	Semimatte
	Cream to powder	Medium/total	Matte
	Pancake cream	Total	Dewy
Sensitive (use oil-free, fragrance-free dermatologically tested makeup)	Liquid	Light	Moist
	Cream to powder	Medium	Matte

forms and shades to meet your every color foundation need. The chart that follows shows the range of foundations available, based on skin type.

Skin Coloring Alternatives

Product research on tinted cosmetics is still limited for African American women. A few exist, and I encourage you to try tinted moisturizers and powders. Tinted moisturizers provide a protective barrier between your skin and the environment. The combination of tinted moisturizer and tinted powder, with tinted lip moisture complemented with a soft brown or black matte eyeliner, and brush-on brow powder and a medium-to-dark cover stick will give you a great semimatte eyelid like many of the famous black actresses and models.

Makeup Finish

Black skin that looks oily and greasy is not attractive when color is applied. Likewise, dry skin can look dull, sallow, and ashen and will lack a healthy luster without a moist finish. If your skin is very oily and you prefer a finish with no shine or sheen, request a matte makeup finish. If you have normal to combination skin, you may desire an ultrasmooth semimatte finish (a slight shine). If your skin is dry, strive for a moist, dewy finish that will give your skin a natural glow.

During extremely hot and humid months (July and August), use three alternatives for relief from very oily skin.

Ways to Deal with Oily Skin

1. Clear skin. Use a light, oil-free moisturizing lotion, with an oil-absorbent, shaded powder.

2. Use an oil-control lotion or blotter, with an oil-control, shaded powder.

3. Problem skin. Skip the moisturizing step and apply an oil-free liquid foundation, since the oil from your skin is usually sufficient. Use a deep-pore cleanser and deep-pore cleansing mask frequently, with fragrance-free, dermatologically tested powder shades.

Beauty Trend Watch

Some cosmetics companies and beauty authorities introduced foundation with the shine look. This is achieved with oil-based, liquid or cream foundations and powders that sparkle and shine.

CREATE YOUR SPECIFIC FOUNDATION LOOK

When you go to a cosmetics counter, especially one in an upscale department store, it is important to inform the beauty adviser or makeup artist what you are looking for and what you can expect from your foundation makeup. There are some specific foundations that can give you a natural or soft velvet look, or can be a foundation for problem skin that will still give you a soft, natural look.

CREATE A BARE HEALTHY-GLOW LOOK

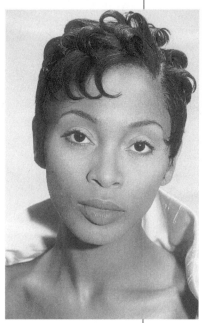

To create a bare healthy glow, you want a foundation finish that is sheer, light in texture, and provides a natural look. If you have normal to combination skin, then a sheer foundation is usually best. You have nothing to hide and have an even-tone skin.

CREATE A VELVET GLOW LOOK

Light to medium coverage is the foundation coverage for the woman with an uneven skin tone, with blemishes, or with dull patchy areas and visible pores. When you use a velvet glow coverage, the skin takes on a very soft, velvet texture.

CREATE A SMOOTH REFINED LOOK

This coverage is perfect when your skin has real problems: stretch marks, dark and light spots, superficial scars, dull sallow places, gray patchy areas, and blemishes. When applied properly, the effect this foundation creates can appear very natural, without a mask-like, heavy, ashen look. (For best results, consult the facial chart in chapter 3 for movement directions.)

I do not recommend color washes, bronzing gels, or tints and color adjusters for black women. To date, not enough research has been done on black skin tones to convince me that these items benefit black skin as they do white skin, for which they were designed. I am not against them, but they have not been color-keyed to the thirty-nine shades of black pigmentation.

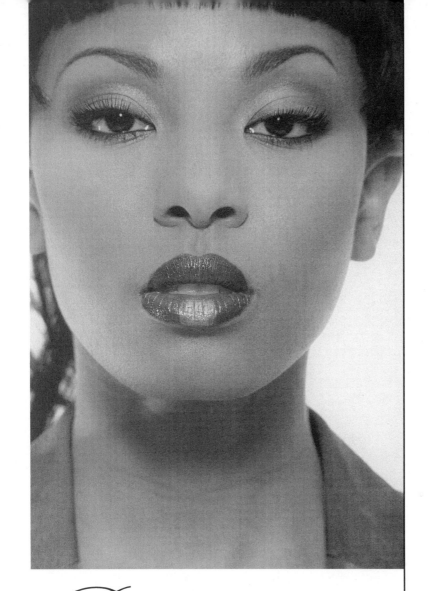

$\mathscr{B}$LENDING YOUR FOUNDATION

13

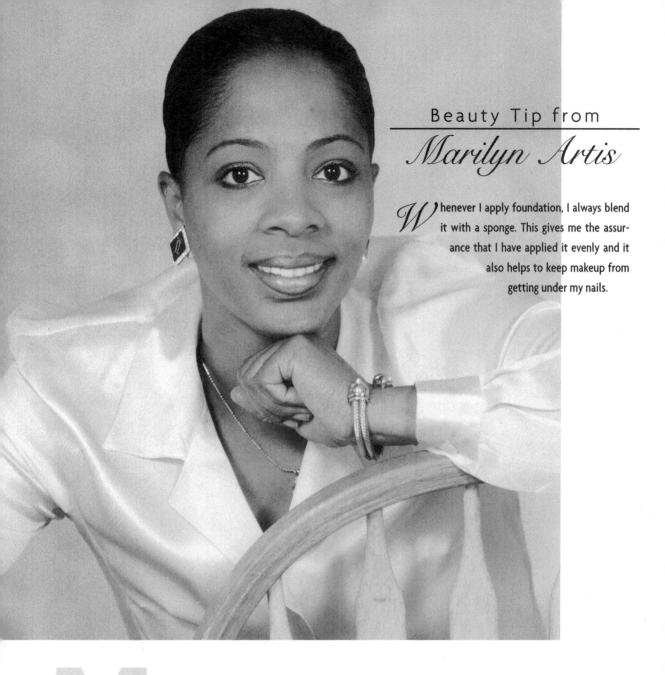

Beauty Tip from
Marilyn Artis

*W*henever I apply foundation, I always blend it with a sponge. This gives me the assurance that I have applied it evenly and it also helps to keep makeup from getting under my nails.

Marilyn Artis, a marketing management specialist, successful entrepreneur, writer, motivational speaker, special events producer, and fashion consultant, is the president of For the People (FTP) Productions. She also writes a weekly advice column for the *Queens Courier* newspaper.

Very few women understand how to apply foundation to get the smooth but natural look they want. For example, many women mistakenly apply foundation most generously to their chin. Instead, they should apply less foundation at the chin area because of the way facial hairs lie on the skin.

Applying your foundation is an art. A common mistake many black women make is to put on too much foundation, believing this is the only way to get total coverage. But the object is to use just enough foundation and to develop a rapid way of getting complete and natural coverage on your face.

Tools

The best tool for applying a soufflé, cream, or pancake cream foundation is a sponge. I am a firm believer in using a sponge. It is clean and it frees the hands; it is better than your fingertips because the warmth of your fingers can cause streaking. But don't wipe your skin with the sponge. Use a press, dab, and pat movement (see the illustration to the right). This allows you to place the proper amount of color where it's needed.

As you know, a sponge has holes, and as you press the sponge onto the surface of the foundation, it lifts away the product. So press quickly, lift quickly, and apply to the face. I don't recommend sponges for applying a liquid foundation, though, because they have a tendency to absorb too much liquid. Once you apply the liquid foundation with your fingertips, however, you can go back over your work with a damp sponge to smooth your foundation to the finish you want.

For those women who use a soufflé with a liquid cream, a cream, or a pancake foundation, the sponge is the best tool for application. The cream stick is another item that can be applied to your face with a sponge.

Many women use a thick, round sponge that's sold at most cosmetics counters. But most women who have spoken to me find

Press, dab, and pat with your fingers, holding the applicator as illustrated. Do not wipe.

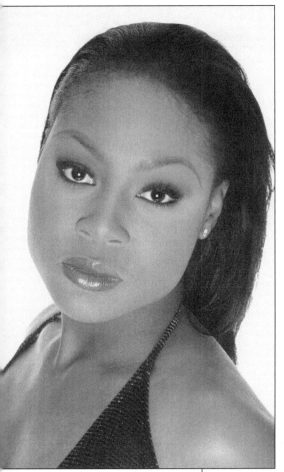

these sponges to be cumbersome. You have to fold them in half and press them to your skin. Sometimes they unfold, slip, crumble, and even come apart. Why use a big sponge when you use only half—and that half with difficulty? Besides, the round sponge is very difficult to clean. There are square sponges, but most women find them too flat and, again, too cumbersome. The ideal sponge is triangular, so that it can be held between the index and middle finger and the thumb. Use a triangular sponge, employing the technique of press, dab, and pat. Don't wipe, scrub, or use a rubbing motion.

PLACING THE FOUNDATION ON YOUR FACE

Where and how you place the foundation is very important. Put one dot on the forehead, one on each cheek, and one on the chin (maybe add one on the tip of the nose, a fifth dot). Use a sponge or your fingertips and blend the dots into one another, working out to the hairline and jawline. If you are using a liquid foundation, place four dots of it on your face, then blend them together. (If you have oily skin and are using an oil-free product, be aware that you must use it rapidly because these products dry quickly—in approximately thirty seconds. If you are too slow, the dots will dry, and you will be able to see where you placed them on your face.)

Once again, think in terms of facial zones. The center zone of your face is called the T-zone, and you should start to apply the foundation here. Begin at the forehead and move toward the temples and around the eye area.

Circle around the eye area, as if to get an owl-eye look. You don't want to put foundation on the eyelids or under the eye—just up to the rim of this area. The reason for using this owl-eye approach is that ingredients in some formulations might affect such sensitive areas.

If you have blemishes in these areas, use a cover stick or a concealer as a foundation for eye shadow and to erase any darkness under the eyes. Remember: your application movements should always be outward toward the hairline, but the stroking, pressing, dabbing, and patting motions are lightly downward. This will encourage any facial hair to lie flat, since hair usually grows downward. Movement then is from the center of the T-zone, blending the forehead, temples, and under the eyes, then moving to the cheeks and then lightly from the cheekbone down toward the jawline.

You should lighten your application when reaching the jawline, so that your foundation blends evenly below the jaw. There should be no demarcation line between the jawline and the neck. You do not—and should not—carry the foundation beneath the chin and jawline onto the throat and neck. I repeat: application is from the center of your face outward toward the hairline. The movements are press, dab, and pat, stroking lightly downward to press the hair down.

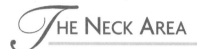HE NECK AREA

For many years I have been against putting foundation on the neck; I am still against it, because there is no reason to do it. When the cosmetics chemist keys color to your facial area, he or she uses the color tones in the center of your face and moves outward toward the hairline to determine your undertone. Colors of black skin vary greatly in terms of shading at the temples, at the center of the face, on the jawline, and on the neck. You can't judge facial color based on the color of your hands, arms, neck, or jaw—they are generally all different. So if you want a true facial color tone, you must go by the suggestions I make for matching skin color to proper foundation.

There are but a few exceptions to what I have just stated. If you have an extremely light face, and it is much lighter than your neck, then select a foundation that is a little darker, so as to match the dark tones of your neck. If your face is darker and neck lighter, then you should choose a foundation just a little lighter. It may look a little strange at the center of your face when you apply it initially, but as you blend the foundation in, you will see how it complements the neck color.

With this method, your facial color, foundation, and neck color will blend. Remember: when someone looks at you, he or she doesn't stare at a particular part of your face or neck unless you do something striking to draw the person's eye. What people do, however, is look at you in a general way. They look for an overall impression. If you make the areas close to the temples and jawline blend with the neck color, whether darker or lighter than your face, you will convey the impression that both are the same color. It is the eyes' impression that you are after.

Another reason why you should not color your neck is that the cosmetics will soil your clothing. I have found this to be a serious problem for so many women who apply foundation or powder to their necks.

Option: for severe neck discoloration, see for alternatives the following discussion on pages 101–104 on the smudge-proof/waterproof color-coded concealers alternatives.

Achieving "Normal Skin"

What you might call "perfect" skin, we in the cosmetics field call "normal" skin. Normal skin is facial tissue with few blemishes and very little roughness or peeling. Many of you may have such skin. Normal skin has a uniform coloration that permits the upper skin layer to admit and reflect light (translucency), with unclogged pores. Some individuals maintain their normal skin all their lives with limited effort. But generally they are the exception. For most people, "normal" skin must be achieved—and it is achievable.

SURFACE SKIN IS THE KEY

It will appear that I am repeating myself, and to some degree I am, but surface skin is the key to a fine appearance. And caring for surface skin can improve it. Clearing the surface of dead cells will improve your skin; under normal conditions, it will perfect the condition of your skin.

Clearing should be done with a mild toner. It actually removes the dead skin, which often is not visible to the eye but gives a look of slight roughness and aging. In contrast, when I mention exfoliating, I refer to an astringent, which some women may need.

IT GETS WORSE BEFORE IT GETS BETTER

If you have neglected your skin—particularly if you have oily skin with subliminal blemishes, blackheads, and whiteheads—your complexion may appear to get worse once you begin taking care of it. You may even find pimples you didn't see before. Don't worry. Your skin is a means by which your body rids itself of impurities. So when you cleanse and improve your system, you may well find your body expelling impurities through its facial pores, and this can result in temporary facial skin problems. Also, what you see on your face may be merely the blemishes becoming more visible as the dead outermost layer is removed. Thus, the blemishes are now closer to the surface and more visible—but also easier to address.

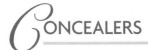# ONCEALERS

YOUR SKIN MAY NEED A CONCEALER

Facial hair is but one skin condition that many women want to alter. Other features you may find disturbing, if not unsightly, are age spots, blemishes, stretch marks, tattoos, birthmarks, varicose veins, and the like.

If this rings true for you, go back to chapter I and read the material on nutrition and your skin. Through good nutrition you can improve the health of your skin and thereby erase, retard, or stop some of these detractions. When this is not possible, or in the interim period during improvement, then your appearance may benefit from cosmetic coverings or concealers. But believe me, you can best improve the basic condition and look of your skin through diet.

USING A CONCEALER

Let's discuss cover sticks (semiconcealers) and concealers themselves below.

COVER STICKS

A cover stick generally comes as a squeezable tube or lipstick-type tube. In either case, you apply the cream to the spot or area you wish to hide. The cover stick is generally for mild pigmentations and discolorations.

Cover sticks are excellent tools borrowed from the theater to conceal certain flaws anywhere on you face, with special consideration for shadows under the eyes, lines around the eyes near the temples, dark eyelids, lines around the nose and mouth, and the cleft in the chin. Cover sticks usually come in beige-yellow tints in light, medium, and dark and are especially blended for black women. If you have a medium-dark skin tone, use a cover stick a shade darker so as not to play up the often lined and puffy tissue. The goal is to give the illusion that where the dark skin, upper lid, and area under the eyes come together is lighter, softer, and therefore smoother than it really is. In most cases, I prefer to apply the cover stick on top of foundation. The creams blend better and the cover stick formula stays put longer because it has something to cling to; also, it won't crease, slip around, or bleed. Use

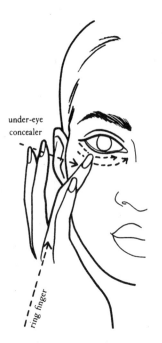

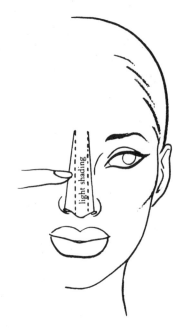

Use your ring finger to apply undereye concealer or cover stick beneath the eye or above the eyelid, moving left to right. The cover stick can also serve as a foundation for eyeshadow.

Apply light cover stick down the center of your nose. Apply darker cover stick or contour powder on each side of your nose, shading the nostril area. Gently blend with your fingertip and set with powder.

your ring finger to gently pat on the cover stick formula, as illustrated above. On dry eyelids, use a cover stick to achieve a smoother finish for your eye shadow and to keep the shadow in place. You can also use a cover stick to contour your nose; see the illustration above.

WHAT IS A CONCEALER?

Most black women are plagued with scars, pigment discolorations, varicose veins, stretch marks, and the like. The cosmetics industry has finally discovered this and has done an outstanding job in now providing quality products for black women with these conditions. Concealers are waterproof cover-ups for large areas.

Several companies have revolutionized the cosmetics industry with their concealing products keyed to the dark pigmentation of African Caribbean,

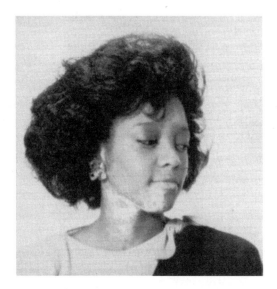 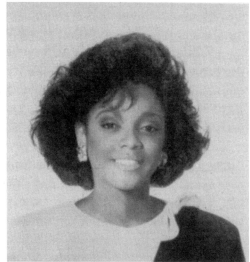

African Latin, African European, and African American women, especially formulated to cover leg veins and stretch marks. Concealing cream shades can blend easily with shades in their liquid, cream, and pancake cream foundations. For all skin types, these corrective creams are waterproof, nongreasy, and smudge free (a plus for oily skin). They easily conceal most skin imperfections, such as scars, burn marks, blotches, blemishes, undereye shadows, age spots, birthmarks, broken capillaries, varicose veins, stretch marks, surgical discolorations, and tattoos. Black women have been waiting for these products for years. I have used concealing creams and corrective creams, and I recommend them highly. The illustration shows how a concealer has been used for vitiligo. Vitiligo is a skin disorder caused by a loss of pigmentation in certain areas, creating "patchy" or light areas on your skin.

There is even a wonderful concealer that is guaranteed to adhere to your skin when properly applied—so much so that you can wear the concealer while swimming and no one will know.

APPLYING A CONCEALER

I will now suggest how to apply a concealer for maximum effect. First, your skin has to be "squeaky clean." The manufacturers supply directions for their products, but they all say basically the same thing: clean skin is a must before application; apply concealer directly to the affected area using a spatula that generally comes with the product; apply the product a little at a time.

If you don't like to use the spatula, use your hands to apply the concealer, but make absolutely sure that both hands are clean. Apply the product with your fingertips and gently spread a light covering over the entire area so that the treated area is indistinguishable in color from the surrounding skin. You may find that by warming the product in the palms of your hands, it can be applied more easily. Always start at the center of the area and move outward. When the concealer completely covers the area, and is properly matched, it will almost melt and blend into your natural color.

While the concealer is still damp, immediately apply the specially formulated powder in order to set, seal, and dry the concealer. All of this must be done before you can touch the area. It shouldn't take more than a minute to apply the concealer and powder. As long as the concealer is applied rapidly and is still damp when you begin with the powder, you are safe.

Now you can decide whether you wish to use a foundation. Most women will. Apply your foundation along the outer edge of the concealed area. Blend it in there and over the rest of your face.

The key to successful use of a concealer is to pair the right concealer and foundation with your skin color. Then you can blend at the edges, or demarcation line, to achieve a flawless look. Your concealer and foundation should be used together. If the concealer and foundation match your natural skin color, you will have no problem following the directions and getting the required coverage.

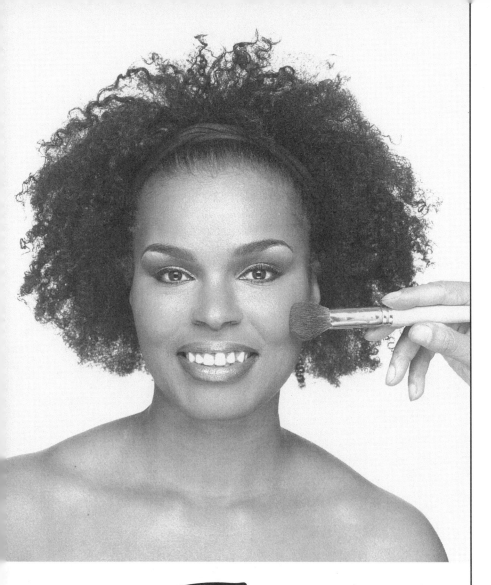

THE BEAUTY OF COLOR–FLAWLESS MAKEUP REVIEW

14

Once you have cleansed, toned, and moisturized your skin properly, you'll be ready to apply foundation and paint your eyes, cheeks, and lips. But in order to achieve a flawless makeup application, you will first need the proper tools.

Your Color Tools

The tools that I discuss here may, in some instances, be different from those you have previously used. However, these are the ones I believe are the easiest and most functional.

powder brush

eye shadow brush

blush brush

brow brush

contour brush

lash comb

eyeliner brush

lip liner pencil

eye shadow sponge

lipstick brush

Having the right equipment is important, but you also must know the proper techniques and procedures for applying your makeup. In the previous chapters we discussed skincare. The next few chapters are about foundations and powders. This chapter is a preview of some of the techniques that you will be able to apply once you have completed this book. I know that many of you have your own techniques and procedures already, but I urge you to compare your methods with what I am about to propose. And for those of you who have no method, or who have been confused by the myriad products available to you, I offer the following steps:

STEPS FOR APPLYING MAKEUP

1. Cleanse.

2. Tone.

3. Moisturize.

4. Apply concealer (optional).

5. Apply foundation or base.

6. Reapply concealer (optional).

7. Apply powder.

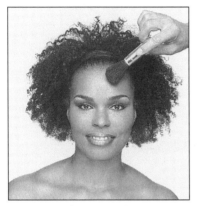

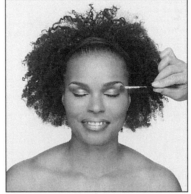

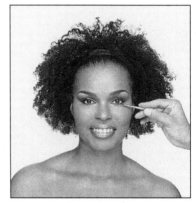

You have set your eye concealer and makeup foundation with powder. Apply your powder before and after (as a finishing powder) eye, cheek, and lip color have been set in place.

APPLYING EYELID COLOR

- Highlight the brow bone and under the eyebrow area.
- Contour the center of the eyelid to give the eye a concave effect.
- Apply fashion color and blend—the key to smooth, natural-looking color.

- Apply liquid, cake, or pencil color. Keep it simple.
- Edge in color, placing line close to upper and lower lashes for drama.

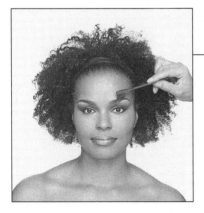

- Apply powder, brush-on-brow, or brow pencil.
- Apply brow gel for ultra brow control, and of course, that natural look and feeling.
- Tweeze, wax, and trim brow for grooming.

Remember, in brushing brow hairs, always move from the center of the face outward toward the temple area.

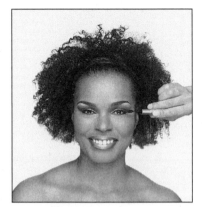 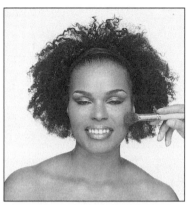 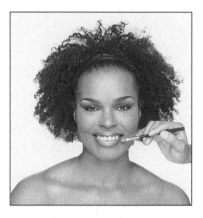

Apply mascara. If lash hairs are semicurled, short, or stubby, then position the wand vertically and swing wand back and forth, touching the tips of lashes. This builds, creating a volumous effect.

Apply blusher for cheekbone highlight.

Apply lip pencil, lip color, and lip gloss, moving with lipstick brush, from corner of mouth toward the center . . . like a real pro!

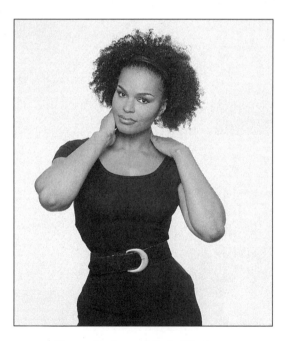

Egypt looks and feels fabulous!

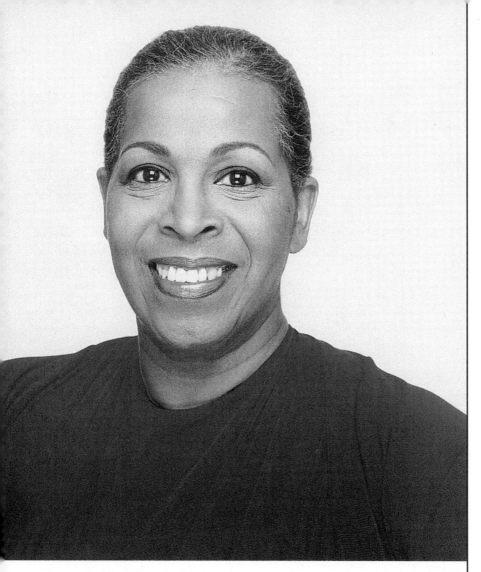

*V*IVA LA DIFFERENCE!
GREAT TRANSFORMATIONS—
A STUDY OF **SKIN**
COLOR AND MAKEUP

15

The four women whom you are about to meet in this chapter fall into the middle range of skin tone complexions. The middle range is the most difficult to match because it is often temporary. For example, women who travel may get a tan in Bermuda or Trinidad. But when they return to a cold climate in Chicago or New York, and their tans begin to fade, they will need different makeup. Not to worry, however. There are numerous companies that have made an excellent effort to match some thirty-nine-plus African American skin tones from the dark end of the spectrum of color to the fair tones of black women worldwide.

These four beautiful women do not have any visible skin problems. Beautiful women they are, indeed. And my team, along with the artistic skills of makeup artist Byron Barnes, made them even more beautiful.

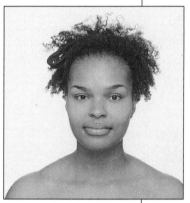 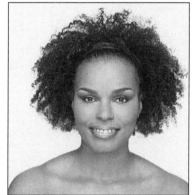

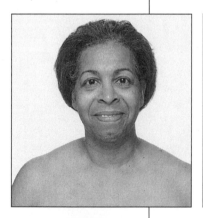 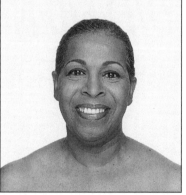

Egypt's undertones are yellow and olive, even though her skin-tone category is medium-dark. Her skin is flawless except for minor blemishes. We applied a cream soufflé in brown blaze glow with complementary transglow pressed powder. Her eyes come alive with winterberry/golden chestnut eyeshadow; cheeks are softly buffed with chocolate chip blusher, and lips are topaz color with a pearl frost.

Elizabeth has a light-to-medium skin tone with yellow undertones and a tinge of olive. She has clear, unblemished skin, perfect for light, cream to powder sand foundation. In fluorescent lighting, her undertones can appear to be flat and lifeless. Her skin tone needs a warm glow, especially during the fall and winter months. However, interestingly, her skin tans to a beautiful bronze glow during the spring and summer months, requiring less foundation. Full lips are still in! I'm sure you will agree, the plum brown lipstick creates a dramatic effect for day or evening. For evening, a light lip frost would bring more pizzazz. A beautiful natural-looking face of color!

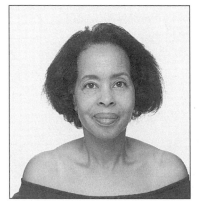 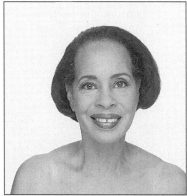

Beverly has clear, smooth, but blemished skin tones. She inherited her natural dark circles and facial flesh moles on the cheek areas. Her undertone is a sallow yellow with a tinge of brown (red). In our search for complementary colors, my team selected the clay cream to powder matte foundation. Eye concealer was applied to the dark eyelids and under the eyes to give a greater effect around the eyes. She has beautiful, radiant eyes and a warm smile. We give definition to her sparse eyebrows. Byron applied powder, brush-on-brows with eyeliner, and a heavy waterproof mascara. Beverly's eyes sparkle with clay, tan, and beige colors; cheeks are brushed with subtle cinnamon color; and lips shine with bronze lipstick over light brown lip pencil and frost lip gloss. She sparkles with the beauty of color!

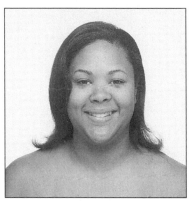

Of Jamaican descent, Nilsa is a newly-wed and Gregory's pride and joy! Young women should be careful not to age their appearance with heavy applications of makeup during the daylight hours. Keeping this in mind, we used crème powder foundation and plum and violet colors on the eyes, cheeks, and lips. Her undertones are yellow/brown (red), which can interfere with inappropriate liquid and crème foundations that have

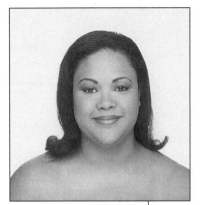

pink or red color in their formulations. The skin's aura is dull and ruddy in appearance. The light beige foundation is perfect for this brown beauty. Nilsa is comfortable with her full figure and aspires to become a full-figured model. She is required to apply makeup to create a little drama, especially around the eyes. The theatrical lighting brings the eyebrow, eyelid, cheeks, and lip definition into focus, accentuating her skin tones. She is a beauty!

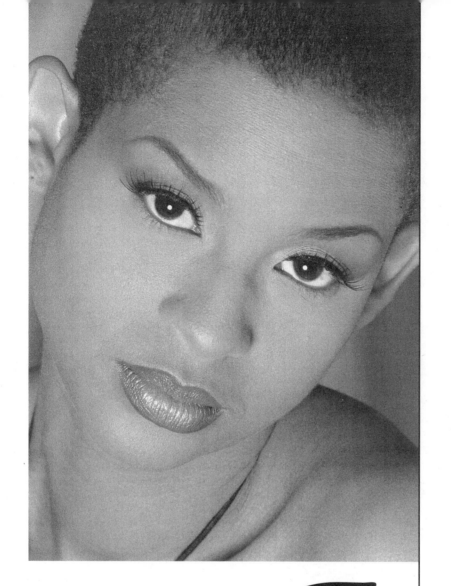

FACE POWDERS

16

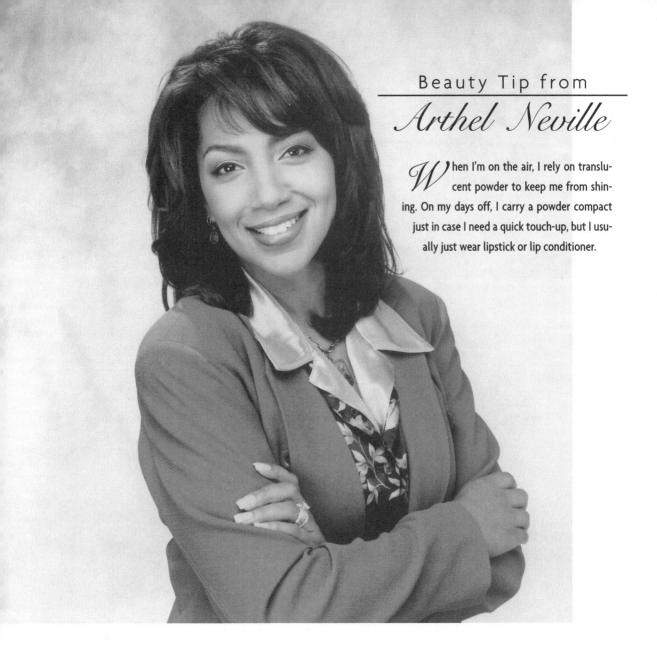

Beauty Tip from

Arthel Neville

When I'm on the air, I rely on translucent powder to keep me from shining. On my days off, I carry a powder compact just in case I need a quick touch-up, but I usually just wear lipstick or lip conditioner.

Arthel Neville launched *Extra,* became a senior correspondent on Fox Files, and then was aboard as an anchor. She is now at the helm of Fox News Channel's entertainment division, anchoring live entertainment updates daily and cohosting the network's entertainment newsmagazine show *Celebrity Spotlight.*

Many black women have decided that they do not need or cannot use powder, largely because they have gotten poor results. However, powder can eliminate the shine for those women whose skin tends to be slightly oily.

Applying powder to your foundation also prepares your face, giving it a silky texture on top of which to apply your blush. However, some makeup artists want you to apply foundation first, other colors next, and powder last, to set the face.

Which method you use depends on your skin type. In deciding when to apply powder I divide black women into two skin types: those with oily skin should apply powder immediately after the foundation; those with dry skin should apply the foundation first, then the eye and cheek color, and set the face with translucent powder. Women with normal skin have the option to use no powder or minimal powder. No special applications are required.

Types of Powder

There are two types of powder, and they have purposes other than that of setting your foundation: translucent setting powders and shaded, or pigmented, powders. Translucent powders are usually loose formulas, with a tint of either amber or bronze. These are usually termed translucent because you can see through the powder to your skin, which will have a glow. These setting powders are used to absorb surface oil and perspiration—for example, for touch-ups before work, after lunch, on the T-zone, and on the cheeks.

I have no problem with black women using shaded powders in place of foundation and translucent powder. Shaded powders are for women who prefer to use a moisturizer and may not use a liquid, cream, or pancake cream foundation. They may be bought either loose or solid in a compact. Shaded powder is applied over your moisturizer and is a pigmented powder.

Remember, though, that pigmented powder not keyed to your foundation coloring can disturb it if worn with foundation. For instance, if you have a

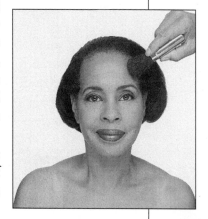

bronze foundation and you put a sable powder over it, the result will be a muddy look, giving a gray, dull appearance to the skin. In contrast, translucent powders need not match your color skin. They are designed to set the foundation and absorb the perspiration and oil deposits associated with the foundation.

You do not have to worry about today's powders lending an ashy or gray look to your skin. When keyed properly, this will not happen. It is titanium dioxide, a white talcum powder, which usually gives that look to black skin. Just make sure the powder you choose is the right color and has been researched for you. Because so many black women have had problems in the past when they used powders designed for white skin, they now use no powder at all. Fear no more! You can achieve wonderful results with powders that are appropriate for your skin.

In summary, some people want to have moist-looking skin while others want a semimatte or matte appearance. Powder should be used for the purposes suggested. If you don't want a shine, use powder. The option is yours.

THE BENEFITS OF POWDER

Today's powders will not dry your skin. Many black women feel that powder causes a gray or ashy look. This is not true. Most powders have some type of moisturizing agent, and the amount depends on the brand. When properly applied, powders will impart a natural, translucent sheen to the face.

It is important that women with black skin use only translucent powder after applying foundation. You don't want to use shaded powders to dust or set your foundation. Also, remember that a little powder goes a long way. You don't need to use a lot of powder to set your foundation. A "cakey" effect is not attractive, and it emphasizes any lines you have under your eyes, around the nose and mouth, and even the cleft of the chin. Think of putting a sheer veil over your face; that is the amount of powder to apply. The ideal is to use powder to set the foundation and to allow the skin and color foundation to glow.

THE BENEFITS OF POWDER

1. Sets makeup foundation.
2. Absorbs oil and perspiration.

3. Does away with the shine.

4. Blushers glide on more easily and set better.

HOW TO APPLY POWDER

Loose powder comes in a container with a scoop-out feature, so it can be reused and so as not to spoil the entire product. A shaker container is ideal for some women; the powder can actually be shaken out of the container. It is like a salt or pepper shaker—you can measure the amount of powder and control its spillage. There is also compact powder. In this instance, you cannot shake or pour the powder, but rather, you use a flat puff applicator to lift the powder from the container to your face.

A cotton ball is usually used to apply loose or pressed powder. A powder puff is usually flat and is used for applying pressed powder. The fluffy powder puff is usually used for loose powder, while the fluffy powder brush, which is an ideal applicator, is highly recommended for applying loose or pressed powder.

HOW TO GET THE LOOK YOU WANT

What look do you want? The matte look is achieved with loose powder and the fluffy puff. Press, dab, and pat is again the operation in applying loose powder (see illustration).

To achieve a sheen (a moist look), again use loose powder, but apply it with a powder brush. To achieve an oil-free, perspiration-free look, women with oily skin, or women who do not want a shine in the T-zone, use pressed powder with a flat puff or a cotton ball. Pressed powder, in general, is ideal for oil absorption; in fact, there are pressed powders designed for oil absorption. You should ask for these particular formulas at your cosmetics counter if you are trying to rid your skin of perspiration and oil.

Once again, let's make sure you understand that there should be no scrubbing, no rubbing. Doing this only takes off your makeup and redeposits it, usually in the very places you don't want it.

Use a powder puff to press, dab, and pat your face with powder, using downward strokes to encourage any fine hairs to lie smooth and even.

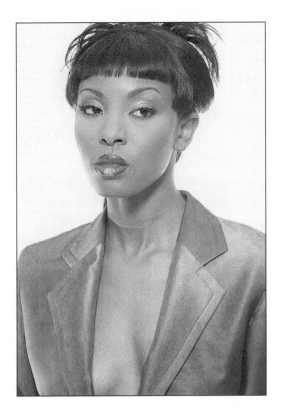

SOME POWDER TRICKS

Use a loose powder whenever you want to take away a line of demarcation. These are usually under the eyes, along the hairline, and on the jawline. Loose powder is excellent for blending your undereye concealer with your blusher. Setting powder can easily be applied between your undereye concealer and blusher to soften the effect, or even erase it, creating a very natural meeting of color.

The trick is to dip the powder brush in the powder and flick away the excess powder, then redip the brush in the loose powder and flip away the loose powder, and then dip the brush into the blusher and shake off the excess. Now you have both the blusher color and the loose powder on the bristles. All you have to do is fan the brush over the line of the demarcation to get a softened effect.

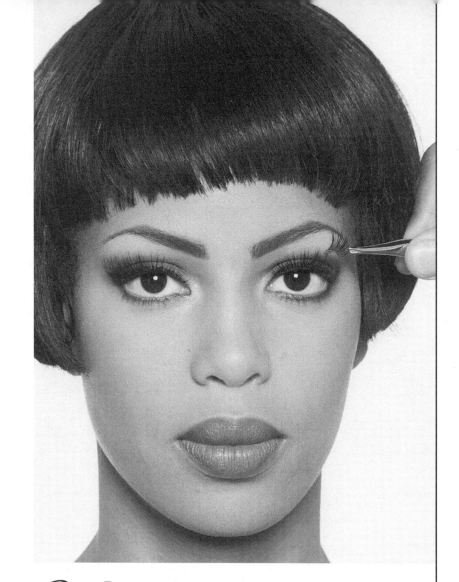

YOUR EYES AND THE USE OF COLOR

17

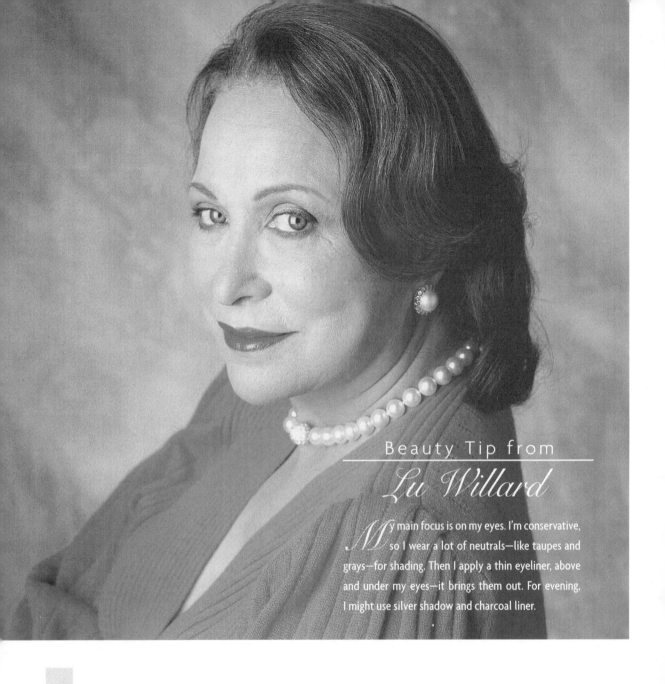

Lu Willard is a highly successful creative design director. She manages marketing, sales, design, and manufacturing for three top jewelry design houses, including suppliers of Kay Jewelers and Macy's.

When I think of eyes, I think of Halle Berry, Mary J. Blige, Brandy, Regina King, Vivica Fox, Lena Horne, Tyra Banks, Pam Grier, Angela Bassett, Vanessa L. Williams, Naomi Simms, Beverly Johnson, Nancy Wilson, and B. Smith—all with eyes that allure, hold, capture, and hypnotize you.

I have had the privilege of designing the eye color for models such as Wanakee, Iman, and Beverly Johnson, and singers Nancy Wilson, Gladys Knight, Melba Moore, and Natalie Cole. The eyes of all these women are beautiful, and their eye makeup enhances their beauty. But the look of each is individual, suited to that person and the world in which she works.

These are the faces of some well-known African American women, and their eyes are made up to hold our attention. Because of this, many black women tend to admire and sometimes yearn to look like these women. I understand this, but I disagree. These beautiful women are made up for the world of films, entertainment, and fashion. What is important is that you not imitate them but find a look that complements *your* lifestyle.

*H*OW TO APPLY EYE MAKEUP

I have designed a simple system for you. It is a four-step, full-scale rainbow eye system in which we consider the correct approach to the eye shape, eyeliner, and lash application. The color chart in the middle of the book will guide you in making appropriate color choices. The major principle is to keep the look clean, blended, and subtle. The exception is with evening makeup, when you should exaggerate to shine and sparkle, when *pizzazz* is the operative word.

THE ORDER FOR APPLYING EYE MAKEUP

1. Eyebrow makeup
2. Eyeliner
3. Eye shadow
4. Mascara

Eyebrow Makeup

Blessed is the woman who does not have gaps and scars in her eyebrows. She does not need eyebrow makeup. If you are one of these women, then all you have to do is groom and shape your eyebrows with a brush.

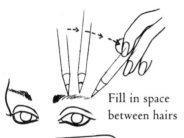

Fill in space between hairs

However, for most women eyebrow makeup fills in the spaces among the hairs and covers any scarring in the brow area.

Eyebrows can easily be filled in with a pencil to give more definition to the line. But don't think in terms of starting at the beginning of your brow and drawing a line to the end, out toward the temples. This is shaping the brow. Below there is an explanation of how to shape the eyebrow by tweezing. But for now you'll just be filling in the spaces among the hairs, according to the existing shape. See the illustration to the left for instructions on filling in sparse eyebrows.

Eyebrow makeup can also be used where you have overtweezed or overplucked. Shape the eyebrow with the pencil and fill in until new growth appears, then do your reshaping. Also, don't be afraid to experiment with the eyebrow. Some eyebrows look great brushed straight up, toward the hairline; just brush them up and fan them out toward the temples. This is a great look, especially for evening.

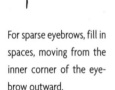

For sparse eyebrows, fill in spaces, moving from the inner corner of the eyebrow outward.

Let's Review

You will need the following tools to shape your eyebrows: tweezers or small round-tip (no points) scissors; brow brush; brow pencil; and alcohol to sterilize after trimming.

How to Shape Your Eyebrow

Step one   Brush brow upward (as I have shown in the past), moving from the center of your forehead toward the temple area—trimming away unwanted individual hairs—following the pencil guideline. Relax and take your time. Brush hairs back in place.

Step two   Still too full and bushy? Brush hairs downward with the brow brush, and move from the center of the bridge of the nose outward to the temple area. This second observation should create a more groomed appearance. Brush hairs back into place.

Step three   Trim away protruding hairs. Use eye makeup remover to wipe away traces of the pencil guideline. A few brow spaces from missing hairs? Fill in with complementary brow pencil, or create a little drama with brush-on brow powder for evening.

EYELINER

Eyeliners come in formulas designed for each skin type and come in different forms: soft pencil, liquid, cream, and pressed cake.

Eyeliners are used to give more definition to the eyes. They highlight the eyes and make the eyelashes appear fuller and thicker. A person can really bring the desired effect to the eyes with a liner; it is the ultimate groomer because it separates the shadow from the lashes via a circle around the eyes.

I think a smoldering and smoky look around the eyes is most attractive on black women, especially darker-skinned women. Eyeliners to some degree have been in disfavor recently because of how they are sometimes worn, giving the eyes a thick and harsh look. But now there are many shades in complementary neutral tones. Rich, deep blues look exceptionally well on black women with medium to dark skin tones. When you use the eyeliner, be sure to color the top lid as well as the bottom.

There is a technique I would like to suggest, especially if you have a problem finding an eyeliner to complement your various shades of eye shadow or your pupils. Take your eye shadow color—maybe the corresponding shade in a dual kit—and simply wet your brush, then stroke the cake of eye shadow for your eyeliner color. For example, if for evening wear you want to use a reddish eye shadow close to the lash, with a dominant red eyeliner that has a little gold in it, moisten your brush and then stroke with the golden-red eye shadow; draw in the color, and presto, you have an eyeliner in a corresponding shade.

PURCHASING YOUR EYELINER

The eyeliner should be color coordinated with your eye shadow. Eyeliners, especially pencils, can be tested on the upper eyelid when you are at the cosmetics counter. Testing foundations as well as eye, cheek, and lip colors is permitted in department stores, chain stores, and some pharmacies. And you should test the colors. Try to test them in natural light, even if you have to stroke the color on your face or eyelid and then excuse yourself to walk to where there is natural light. If you use your makeup mirror to look at the color on your skin, you will see that in different lighting the shades appear differently.

Just a few words of caution. There are waterproof eyeliners that tend to be a little rubbery, but they are excellent if you perspire heavily, if your skin is oily, or if you go swimming a lot. However, I have found that when used frequently these waterproof eyeliners can actually dry out the area around your eyes, leaving it sensitive. This is especially true for those who suffer from allergies or who are naturally sensitive in this area. If this describes your situation, then I suggest you avoid the waterproof eyeliners.

PENCIL VERSUS LIQUID EYELINERS

Liquid eyeliner is still one of the most popular forms, but I recommend the pencil eyeliner because you can control it better. Pencils come in more colors, they can be smudged on the top and bottom of the eyelids; and they can be applied either thickly or thinly. If you have had very little practice applying liquid eyeliner, you can easily lose control. Yet both forms are serviceable and you can have attractive results.

*E*YE SHADOW

For a basic eye color effect, apply highlighter, contour, and then fashion shade.

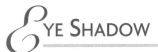

Highlighter

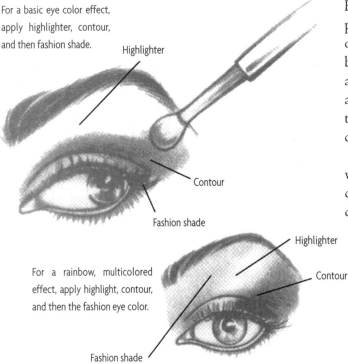

Contour

Fashion shade

For a rainbow, multicolored effect, apply highlight, contour, and then the fashion eye color.

Highlighter

Contour

Fashion shade

Eye shadow comes in cream, crayon, powder, or liquid. The powder shadows are ideal for most skin types because they can be controlled easily and they appear to be softer, silkier, and smoother on your skin. However, the powders are best suited for oily, combination, and normal to oily skin.

The cream shadows are best for women with very dry eyelids. The only caution is that women with medium to dark skin tones should stay away from creams that have a silver or white talc base, since these shadows give the eye area an ashen look. The light materials play up the gritty, chafed areas and dry lines of your eyelids.

The crayon shadows are excellent for smoothing on and blending. They can be very soft, and that is the caution for those of you who have oily skin. Make sure you don't overuse an oil-based crayon shadow, for it can build up a crease and melt on the eyelids.

There are several cosmetics companies that encourage customers to dampen their powder eye shadows because dampening the shadow creates a different consistency and helps it glide on evenly, dry well, and stay put. The instructions ask you to moisten the eye shadow in its dual kit with an eye shadow brush or sponge, and to stroke the eye shadow onto the eyelid so it will dry to a very soft color. The color remains true and stays put, without the creasing so often seen when a cream or liquid shadow is used. The technique is excellent for oily skin.

There are fragrance-free eye shadows for those of you who have sensitive eyes or tend to have an allergy-prone eye area. There are eye shadows that are sold as dual kits: two pans containing two colors that usually are a highlighter and a fashion shade, which can also be used for contours. Then there are four-pan color kits: highlighter, contour, and a fashion shade in a light and a dark hue. You can even find six- and twelve-color pan kits that permit you to mix and blend shades to come up with original colors for a rainbow eye, smoldering eye, or contour eye. Contour shades usually come in neutral colors like cocoa or light brown, or in shades of gray and in the berry shades.

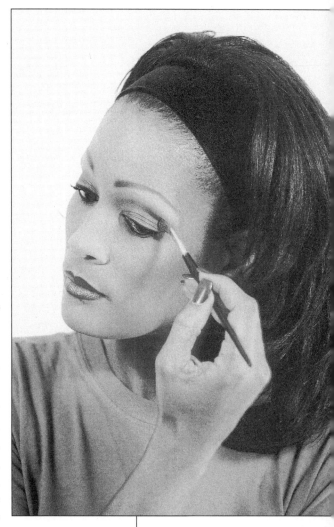

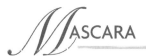ASCARA

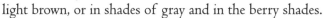

The purpose of mascara is to build up your lashes. Mascara makes your lashes look longer, thicker, and more smoldering. There is a formulation that comes as a cream, which I recommend. For application, see the following illustrations.

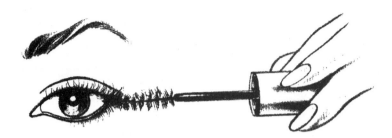

For women with semistraight lashes, hold the brush horizontally and do entire lash, outward and upward, rolling the wand for fullness.

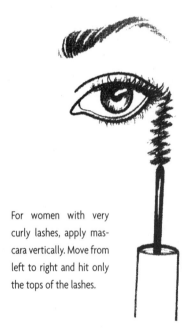

For women with very curly lashes, apply mascara vertically. Move from left to right and hit only the tops of the lashes.

The shades that look best on black women are black, brown/black, dark brown, antique bronze, and berry shades, the newest entries on the market. Don't be turned off by the color intensity in the tube. When applied, these berry shades look very soft around the eyes. In fact, the raspberry, cranberry, green, and navy blue shades look fabulous, day or night.

Don't be reluctant to try colorful mascara. Many white women are discouraged from using these colors during the day, but on professional black women they look excellent anytime. They give a soft and handsome look to the eyes. Pay attention to your mix of colors when you make up, though. Be careful about what color eye shadow you use with a colored mascara. There should be some coordination between the colors of the lashes and the eyelid itself.

Remember to test the mascara before you buy, but don't allow the beauty adviser to apply it from the tester wand directly to your eyelashes. This tester wand has been used on other women, and any bacteria it picked up from them is in the tube. Bacteria grow extremely fast in the dark, warm tubes on the lighted cosmetics counter. That tester wand could put bacteria on your eyes, so make sure you get a clean wand. Cosmetics companies provide disposable wands for testing purposes.

GET THE RESULTS YOU WANT FOR FABULOUS EYES

To make your eyes less round

Liner. Draw a thin line at just the very outer corner of the upper lid and across the bottom lid.

Shadow. Use lots of color, edging shades into contour crease, shading up and out at the corner.

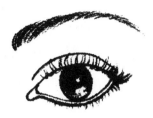 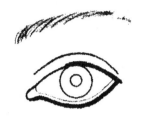 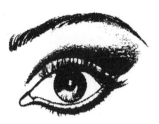

To make your eyes more prominent

Liner. Draw a line from the center of the upper lid out toward the corner. Add a line across the bottom lid.

Shadow. Add a light color to the eye bone, contour color in crease, and use a frosted or light shade on the lid.

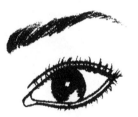 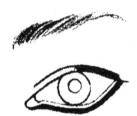 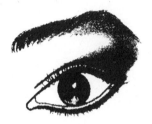

To make your eyes look deeper

Liner. Draw eyeliner across the top lid and from the center to the outer corner. Apply mascara.

Shadow. Add lots of color in the contour crease. Do not apply light frosted shades.

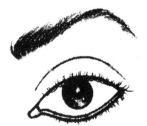 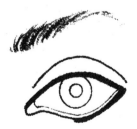 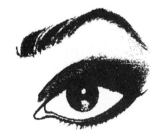

To make small eyes look larger

Liner. Circle the top and bottom inner lids with soft black, deep blue, or rich deep brown. All three colors will make the white of the eyes appear even whiter and the eyes appear wider. Apply mascara.

Shadow. Color is applied to the eye bone under the brow arch, fanning out toward the temples. Contour color in crease and along the lid as illustrated.

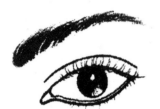 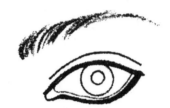 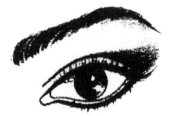

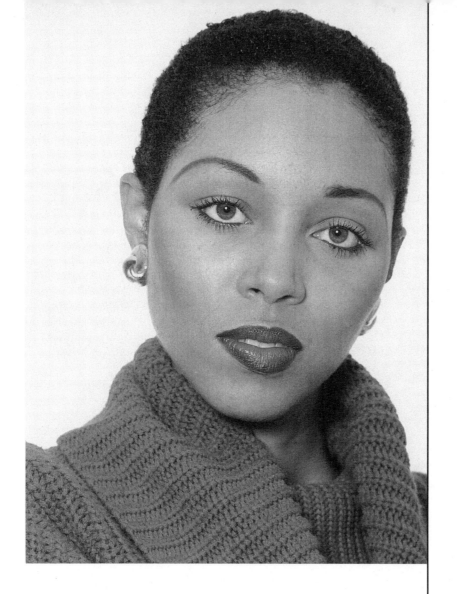

BLUSHERS 18

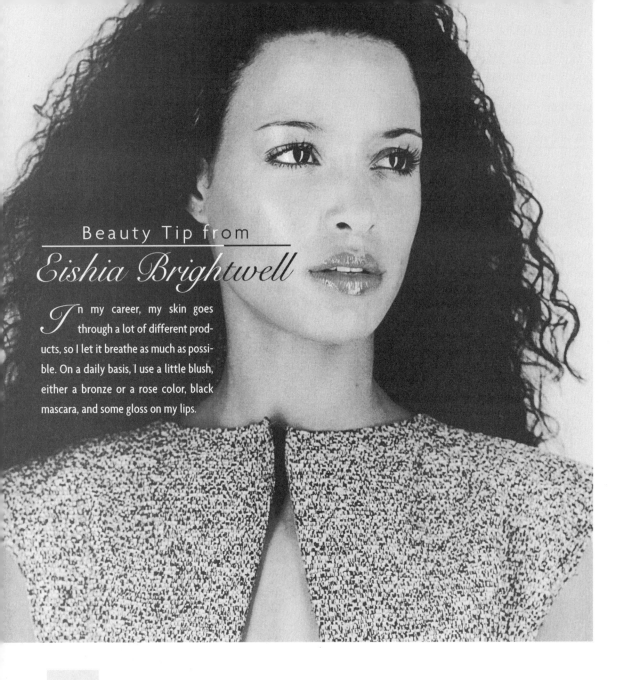

Beauty Tip from
Eishia Brightwell

In my career, my skin goes through a lot of different products, so I let it breathe as much as possible. On a daily basis, I use a little blush, either a bronze or a rose color, black mascara, and some gloss on my lips.

Eishia Brightwell has been modeling since the tender age of eight and has appeared in countless catalog and print ads. She has worked with the famed Wilhelmina Agency in Miami and is now modeling full-time in New York City.

The purpose of a blusher is to bring a blush and a glow to the cheeks. I recommend using blushers because they bring a vibrancy and an alive quality to your face. But you must carefully select the color and place it correctly.

Don't be dissuaded from using blusher because you see intense color compacts on display at retail cosmetics counters. They are usually very bright, but you will be surprised how, when keyed to your skin color, those deep, rich pigmented blushers bring a soft natural glow to your cheeks.

You have probably heard the cosmetics trade call their blusher colors mahogany, golden bronze, loganberry, raspberry, topaz, ruby, ginger, gold, cinnamon, and brown. These are the names of just a few of the blusher products produced. Cosmetics companies have recently developed for blacks many natural, warm, and sophisticated deep-pigmented shades for black skin, which have proved to be excellent.

Your lipstick and blusher do not have to match; however, they should be of the same color family or in the same color range. For example, a red-brown blusher enhances a yellow-based red lipstick. For evening, a true red blusher with golden highlights makes a wonderful partner to a gold-frosted red lipstick with a golden gloss. With this combination your cheeks and lips will be all aglow with golden sparkle, reflecting light against your dark skin. Consult the color chart in the middle of the book for more blusher-lipstick combinations.

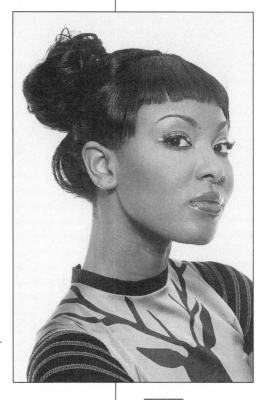

*T*YPES OF BLUSHERS

There are many kinds of blushers sold that create different effects and are made for different skin types. See the table on page 132 for information on each. Here, I discuss two major types of blushers: powders and creams.

POWDER BLUSHERS

Powder imparts a natural-looking, soft-matte finish. Of all the formulas, it is the easiest to apply and looks the best on black skin. Powders glide on smoothly and don't leave a bumpy, ashen buildup. Literally hundreds of powder blushers are available, tailored for every skin type. If you try a blusher that gives a gray appearance to your skin, you can be sure it was not designed for your skin coloring. All skin

TYPES OF BLUSHERS

TYPE OF BLUSHER	FINISH	COVERAGE	TYPE OF SKIN	HOW TO APPLY
Gel tint	Smooth sheen, gold-frosted gels look great at night; don't ever wear frost during the day	Sheer, light texture; should not be deeply pigmented	Combination to oily (most are oil free and water based); not advised for very dry skin; can appear shiny and slick	Use fingertips, on top of foundation, before powder; dry-down period is extremely fast, so you have to work quickly; gel can streak and blotch
Liquid	Moist and smooth	Sheer, light to medium texture; deeply pigmented	All skin types; best suited for combination, medium to dry skin	Use sponge, sliding on top of foundation, then set with powder; easy to apply
Mousse	Soft, dewy-looking; gold-frosted is good at night	Sheer; foam is light textured; not deeply pigmented	Not for dry skin; for oily or combination skin	Use fingertips; blend with a sponge, especially around the edges
Cream	Smooth, dewy; gold-frosted is excellent, some even appropriate for day; best for evening wear; silver-frosted is out forever!	Medium; deeply pigmented; should not ever appear greasy or slick	Normal to dry skin; oil free best suited for oily skin only	Use fingertips and blend on top of foundation, set with powder
Powder	Matte or semimatte frost; gold-frosted is best to highlight cheekbones at night	Medium; deeply pigmented	All skin types; oily skin benefits the most	Use brush

types can wear powder blusher; however, they are best for those with combination or oily skin. Women with sensitive skin must be very careful and use only blushers designed for sensitive skin (usually fragrance- and oil-free formulas).

CREAM BLUSHERS

There are two basic cream blushers—regular and oil free—and they come as a swivel stick or in a compact. Use your fingers or the swivel stick for best application. Apply the cream over your foundation and then add your translucent powder. In general, cream blushers are easy to blend, but avoid the pale shades, red to pinks, and peachy to orange colors, because they appear to be suspended in air or to sit on top of the skin.

Cream blushers are best for combination or dry skin. Oily skin collects the shine and high humidity, and in the summer months the cheeks appear greasy and slick, which is not attractive at all! All skin types should stay away from the frosted cream blushers unless the frost is gold, not silver. I don't think silver enhances medium to dark complexions and it should never be used on the cheeks.

How to Use Blusher

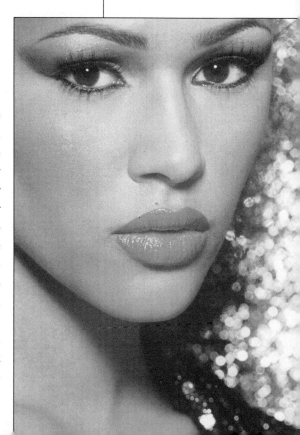

USE WITH MODERATION

Many women wear too much blusher during the day. The ideal application is only a suggestion, or hint, of color. Select rich, pure colors such as copper-bronze with its deep gold base, or a soft plum, light wine-burgundy, or a deeply pigmented almond-orange shade. When you apply powder blusher, always dip the brush quickly and flick or twist your wrist to stroke the cheek lightly. Remember: it is better to apply just a little blusher and then go back and apply more if you need it, than to apply too much and have to disturb the foundation to remove the excess. Matte colors (no shine) are best for day on all skin types. For the evening, gold essence, frosty, and shimmery shades are best.

Generally, I don't recommend stripping, or streaking, even though it is very popular. However, it might work rather well in the evening to create a dramatic effect. Stripping is a theater technique transferred to retail cosmetics. The aim is to have the skin look as though it had been drenched or kissed by the sun, and the effect is achieved by streaking the color at the temples, cheeks, tip of the nose, and chin. Usually it doesn't work. You have to be very good and have a very light touch. It works best, if at all, on white skin. And unless you live in California, Florida, or another sunny climate, it won't look real.

Color Placement

The cheek, according to your facial shape and size, is where you should place the blusher. Don't place it on the nose. After all, why put blusher where it will make you look like you have a cold?

The outer corner of your eye is your guideline for application. Don't ever bring the color toward the broad nostril of your nose; it will ring and broaden your facial structure. Likewise, blusher should not ever be shaded down past the tip of your nose. Draw an imaginary line from the tip of your nose, under your natural cheekbone, to the middle part of your ear; this is usually where you should cut off the shading. Also, most women have a convex eye area, so don't bring the blusher too close to the outer eyes. When applied close to the eyes, blushers tend to make them look puffy and drawn.

Consult the color chart in the middle of the book and the recommendations of the cosmetics company.

No blush zone

Special Blusher Tips

For the ultimate, long-lasting glow, apply a cream blusher over your foundation and set it with translucent powder. Then apply a complementary powder blusher over the translucent face powder and blend. You will have a day-long natural glow.

Contouring or shading your facial features is the easiest way to slim down the face and redefine flawed features.

Special Tips

1.   Use the outer corner (A) as a guide to start adding blusher.
2.   Never apply blusher in the "No blush zone." (B)
3.   Always move across, upward, and out toward the hairline. (C)
4.   Do not add blusher underneath the eyes near the lower rim. (D)

On the top side, apply the radiant, vibrant blusher with your brush sweeping across the cheekbone, blending upward to top of ear.

Use your contour brush and apply a rich matte brown on the bottom side of your cheekbone, moving upward toward the center part of your ear.

For that special glow at night, apply golden powder blusher on temples, between the eyes, on tip of nose, and at base of chin.

Use your contour brush to de-emphasize a full or square chin with a matte brown blusher.

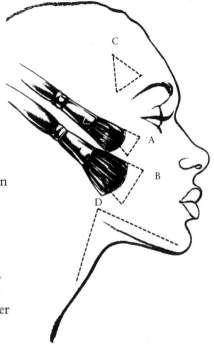

*D*o You Know Your Face Shape?
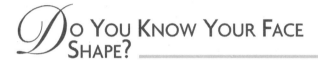

Blushers can do more to add warmth and radiance than any other cosmetics. We feature the following four basic face shapes; however, different faces require different techniques. If your face shape is not here, combine the features from others to obtain the right techniques.

To find your face shape, tie your hair up and away from your face and look into the mirror. If you still can't tell, get a ruler and measure your forehead from temple to temple, cheekbone to cheekbone, and jawline to jawline. Place measurements on paper and connect with rounded lines.

Square Face

You have a firm structure, usually a wide forehead, cheeks, and jawline. The apple, or round part of the cheekbone, registers near the outer corner of your eye. Begin the blusher application at this point, sweeping the cheek color upward to the center part of the ear.

To soften a wide and square face, apply cheek color at the bottom side of the jaw, with the cheekbone, to accent the center of your face. Don't ever apply blusher between the "no blush zone" apple of the cheekbone and the bloom of the nostril.

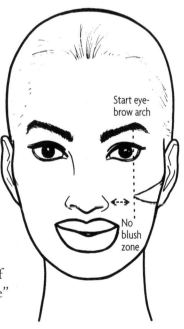

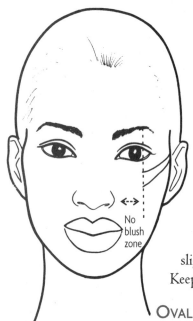

Your eyebrows are most important. No straight, thin lines. Arch your brows at the corner of the pupil so that, looking straight into the mirror, they are in line with your cheekbone.

ROUND FACE

You have a solid, structured face. Keep color high on the cheekbones, sweeping it outward and upward to the top of the ear and hairline. Don't ever place color on the apple and never bring color from the apple toward the bloom of the nose.

You want to discourage a clownish appearance. Sweep blusher from the outer corner of the eye, fanning upward. The eyes are the focal point. Shading is also appropriate at the temples.

Eyebrows should be naturally full and shaped horizontally, with a slight curve. The rainbow eye, placed diagonally, plays down circles. Keep lip pencil line faint and inside the natural lip line.

OVAL FACE

You have the so-called balanced facial structure. Polish the cheekbone with rich, radiant color, sweeping from the outer edge of the corner of your eye and creating a V effect. The open part of the V spreads wide toward the ear and hairline.

Play up the apple, moving straight across and fanning outward. Eyebrows take on a subtle half-moon shape. Accentuate the crease and create a more concave illusion. Highlight with glossy mascara.

Place shading color at the temples, on the tip of the nose, and at the chin. Lips are shaped, moist, and dewy.

NARROW FACE

You have a slim, delicate structure. Start your blusher placement at the outer edge of the apple. Keep color on the cheekbone, toward the top. Make wide sweeps toward the upper part of ear and hairline.

You want to create optical and aesthetic horizontal lines of color to suggest width. Don't shade or contour the temples, jaw-line, or chin. Color in the center zone of the face is important.

Eyebrows should be on a horizontal plane, with a high center arch. Eye shadow is earthy, gold, topaz, peachy red, soft berry. Do not use brown-black or black outer corner shading. Lip pencil liner emphasizes, broadens, and plays up full lips. Apply color to the very edge.

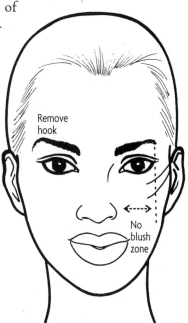

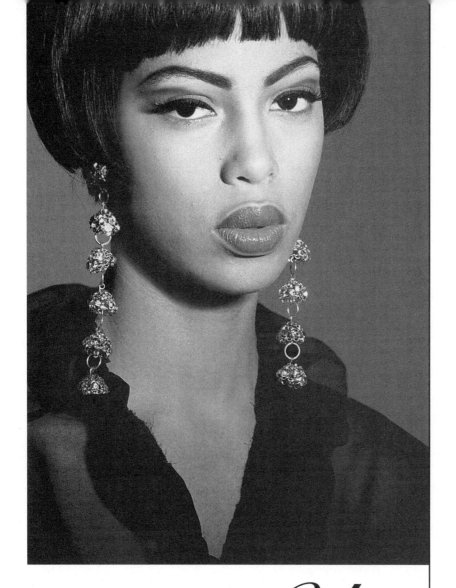

Your Fabulous LIPS

19

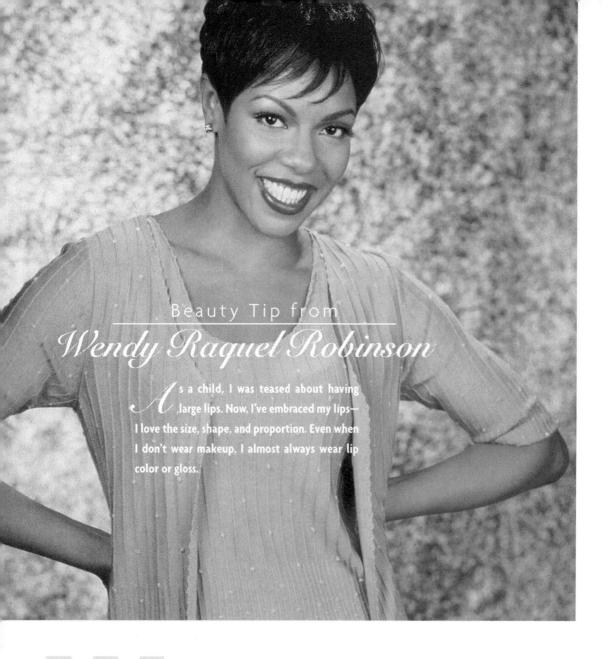

Beauty Tip from
Wendy Raquel Robinson

As a child, I was teased about having large lips. Now, I've embraced my lips—I love the size, shape, and proportion. Even when I don't wear makeup, I almost always wear lip color or gloss.

Wendy Raquel Robinson has found success in the theater as a versatile actress, dancer, singer, writer, and choreographer, and in film and on television, where she stars as a series regular on *The Steve Harvey Show*. Robinson also cofounded Amazing Grace Conservatory (A.G.C.), a theatrical training institute in Los Angeles, where she is the artistic director.

The most attractive part of an African American woman's face is her lips. No one smiles with such full lips and with such beautiful white teeth. The secure black woman who really believes that black is beautiful has no problem accepting God's gift. She flaunts her full lips when talking with a friend, communicating at work, attending religious affairs, flirting, or just being sensual.

A black woman has a natural, firm, raised lip line. The natural pout in the center and her thick upper and lower lips are attractive. Learn how to express your lovely features by practicing before a mirror. Maximize the value and beauty of your lips. But be honest with yourself too. If your lips have droopy, turned-down corners, teach yourself to hold the corners up. Smile more and practice looking pleasant.

Besides how you hold your lips, your mouth may have other "spoilers" needing attention—for example, missing teeth, gold teeth, yellow teeth, or poorly manufactured partial dentures. Your lips dramatically outline your mouth, therefore your teeth must not be a major negative to an otherwise beautiful face. When you have moist, dewy, luscious lips, your teeth in their whiteness and evenness only make you more inviting. Your lips, teeth, and smile make your face radiant, bringing joy to all who see you.

LIP COLOR OPTIONS

If you are a woman who prefers just a hint of natural color (earth tones to soft beige, or pink tones), I have a suggestion: even out discolorations with concealer or your foundation base and set with powder. If your upper and lower lips are dark and even, for best results select a lip shade lighter than your lips.

You might wish to apply a lipstick product from a tube, wand, pan, or pot. There are lip glosses designed for African American women—in deeply pigmented colors—that can be worn alone; they impart a moist, sheer sheen to your lips. Or you might wish to wear a clear lip gloss or lip moisturizer. This, too, would be appropriate. Don't use greasy, nonpenetrating petroleum jelly, however. It looks and feels tacky on your lips. You might want to take the time to use a lip pencil, which is an excellent tool for achieving a natural look. If you use a lip pencil, lightly line the lip and fill in with the pencil, covering any uneven tones, then apply a clear red, a brown lip shade, or clear tint gloss.

If you are conservative but want a pulled-together look, I suggest the medium-tone creams (clear red, russet-red, radiant red, cocoa-copper, cinnamon, café, brandied coral, raspberry, spice sienna, and so on).

Black skin usually looks best in shades of beige, yellow, yellow-brown, and blue. But consult the color chart in the photo insert before selecting a lipstick. For example, if you are of medium tone with yellow-brown skin and a sallow aura, lipsticks with a beige or deep yellow base will drain color from your skin. On the other hand, you can wear deep orange shades such as cinnamon-orange, burnt orange, radiant red, bronze-coral, and claret.

$\mathcal{L}$IPSTICK TOOLS

Now let's consider the lipstick tools and materials: lip liner pencil, lip brush, lip light, lip toner or foundation, and lip balancer.

1. *Lip Liner Pencil.* Liner pencils define the line of the lips and should be chosen with your skin tone in mind. For example, if you have fair to light skin, your liner should be rose-pink, light red, light plum, or light brown. Women with medium skin tones look best using liner pencils in shades of red, light brown, brown, and plum. Those with dark skin tones look best using red, deep brown, raspberry, plum, or brown-black liners. Never use a black pencil to line your lips. It's unattractive and appears harsh.

    When you want a new look for your lips, use a lip pencil to outline it. Lightly outline the lips and fill in the corners if your lips are full, and then edge in your selected color. The pencil should match as closely as possible the desired lip color.

    Black women often have deep folds in their lips that extend to the outer edges. Lip color frequently cakes and peels to these edges, giving the appearance of bleeding color. The lip liner pencil keeps lip color from bleeding and gives a more precise lip line. When matte, oil-free pencils are used as a base for cream or frosted lipsticks, the color stays put and wears much longer.

2. *Lip Brush.* The purpose of a lipstick brush is to transfer lipstick from the tube to the surface of the lips in a smooth application. Most black women have very deep folds, or lines, in their lips. When lip-

stick is applied directly from the tube, the tube rides over the deep folds. The lip brush prevents this from happening, because, owing to its flexibility, the brush gets color into the crevices as well, giving a smooth, full-color application. The lipstick brush also gives you the option of lining your lips (see previous item), reducing the possibility of your lipstick bleeding once the large area is colored.

A lipstick brush may be either man-made, of natural fibers, or a combination of both. I prefer a blend of natural and man-made fibers.

3. *Lip Light.* A lip light is a lip color adjuster, which reflects light colors away from ruddy, bluish, or very dark lips; it is worn under the lipstick.

4. *Lip Toner.* A lip toner, or foundation, is a lip adjuster that corrects slightly discolored lips, evens out lip tones, and keeps color true. Toners come in fair-to-medium and medium-to-dark shades.

5. *Lip Balancer.* A lip balancer is a deep, waxy, purplish-teak natural pigment, designed to camouflage the resistant light pink discoloration often found on medium and dark lips. A lip balancer also neutralizes the acidity that causes discoloration in the center of the bottom lip, an area that is more often affected than the upper lip. In the process, it prevents the lipstick from changing color when placed on this area. A lip balancer is worn under the lipstick. It is excellent for subtle, medium, and deep shades of lipstick; however, the bright reds, orange-browns, and light berry shades are affected by a lip balancer.

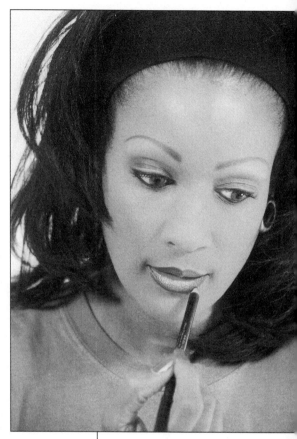

*T*YPES OF LIPSTICK

Choosing a lipstick is a very personal preference, and it is up to you to make that selection. Lipsticks with specially formulated conditioners, moisturizers, waxes, and light mineral oil are superior to those without them, since these ingredients smooth the lips, help retain moisture, help prevent infection, and often protect sensitive skin.

BEAUTY TREND WATCH

Most lipstick formulas include conditioners and emollients. For example, lip moisturizers often contain PABA (a sunscreen) along with vitamins A and E. So there are advantages over and above beauty for using a lipstick.

Now, let's review some of the major types of lipstick available today:

1. *Cream Lipsticks.* Standard cream lipsticks are deep pigment colors without shine. They wear longer and impart more coverage than the noncream sticks, owing to their heavy wax base. A second cream formula is more lightweight in texture and does not feel as heavy on the lips, but it also does not wear as long because it usually has a mineral oil base.

2. *Frosted Lipsticks.* Frosted lipsticks are usually heavy pigment colors with an iridescent, pearlized, or opaque gold coverage. Black women look best in iridescent gold eye shadow, highlights, blusher highlights in gold, and most certainly lipsticks with a gold or a yellow base.

3. *Silver Sparkling Frost.* This usually looks ridiculous if applied to dark or very dark skin. This is because it imparts an ashy-gray look to red-brown or bluish brown skin undertones. I frown on using silver frost, the same way beauty professionals discourage blue eye shadow for white women.

4. *Long-Lasting Lipsticks.* There are lipsticks formulated to last far longer than regular lipsticks. New research and development has produced long-wearing, nonsmear lipstick formulas approved for women of color.

5. *Matte Lipsticks.* No-shine lipstick formulas have conditioners for a nondry look and feel.

6. *Translucent Lipsticks.* Translucent lipsticks in tubes or wands impart just a hint of color, with sheer coverage.

7. *Lip Glosses.* Glosses have a clear, shiny, transparent base. They come in pans, pots, wands, and tubes. Some have conditioners and moisturizers and claim healing properties. They are usually worn over lipstick to impart a sheer gloss. Lip glosses can be worn alone, as well.

8. *Nonfragrance Lipsticks.* Fragrance-free lipsticks are for sensitive and acne skin. Some women may have an allergic reaction to their lipstick and experience swelling or an itchy, burning sensation on their lips. Most women sensitive to lipstick are reacting to the lanolin, fragrance, dyes,

or preservatives in the formula. If this is a problem for you, buy fragrance-free, dermatologically tested, hypoallergenic lipstick.

Applying Lip Color

Most of us have lined, curved, crinkly lips. For best results, edge in a faint lip line with a lip brush or a lip pencil. Buy a shade darker (light and medium brown, red, and berry hues) for aesthetic illusions.

The lip brush is used to pick up a small amount of lip color, and then to outline the lips, filling in from the center of the mouth to the outer edges. The following is the procedure I suggest for having beautifully colored lips.

Technique for Applying Lip Color

1. Apply a lip color adjuster, such as a lip light.
2. Outline your lips with a sharp lip liner pencil.
3. Edge in the lipstick color along the pencil outline and coat the lips, starting with the bottom and moving to the upper lip. Apply more color in the center, moving outward to the edges. If your lips are smooth, apply color directly from the tube.
4. Add lip gloss for a moist effect or a gleam.

See the illustrations that follow for specific techniques.

Full, Puckered Lips with Lines

Your full lips usually have an attractive ridge that gives them a definite lip line. Cover your lips with foundation, preferably an oil-free formula. Blot with oil-free setting powder.

Thin Lips

Cover the lips and edges with foundation. Set with oil-free powder. Redefine the lip shape you want with a lip liner pencil in a shade darker than your selected lip color. Fill in with lipstick and add a touch of gloss to give a moist, dewy appearance.

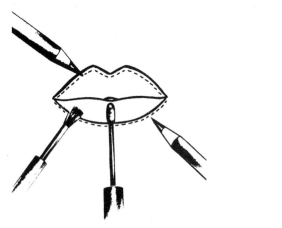
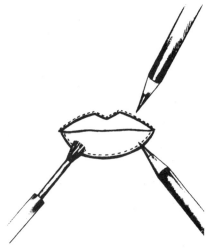

LIPS THAT ARE DIFFERENT SIZES

When one lip is larger than the other, apply foundation over the larger lip, set with oil-free powder, then edge in a line inside your natural lip line with a pencil or brush. Fill in with lipstick. Now follow the natural lip line of the smaller lip with a pencil or brush, and fill in with lipstick.

UNBALANCED AND DROOPY LIPS

Cover the uneven lips with foundation, and set with oil-free powder. Balance the uneven lip portion by straightening the lip line with a pencil, using a shade darker than your selected lipstick color.

DROOPY CENTER

To balance a droopy center, apply medium shade of oil-free concealer vertically through the center of the droop. Outline with pencil and lip brush, and fill in with lipstick. To cover the natural lip line at the corner, edge in with a medium to dark oil-free cover stick. Blot with powder.

Droopy center

Droopy corners

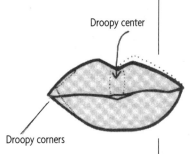

LIFT A CORNER

To lift a corner to create an optical illusion, use a lip pencil to extend the lower lip, taking the line upward. Continue the line just a bit above the upper lip corner.

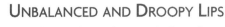

Now, extend the upper lip line to meet it. Blot with powder and fill in with lipstick color.

DISCOLORED LIPS

You have four options for alleviating this problem.

TECHNIQUES FOR HELPING DISCOLORED LIPS

1. Use a lip light to reflect light evenly away from uneven dark lips.

2. Use an oil-free lip toner or foundation to even out lip color.

3. Use a lip balancer as a natural stain to even out and build up on the pink discoloration. A lip balancer will interfere with a light lipstick shade and is not recommended in this instance.

4. Use a medium to dark oil-free cover stick to help even out discolored lips.

DRY, CRINKLY, LINED LIPS

Condition lips with gloss or lip moisturizer, which contains mineral oil, cocoa butter, phenol, alum, camphor, and beeswax. Ask your beauty adviser or read the labels yourself to find out if, indeed, lip moisturizers, lip balm, lipstick, and lip glosses have SPFs of 25 or 30.

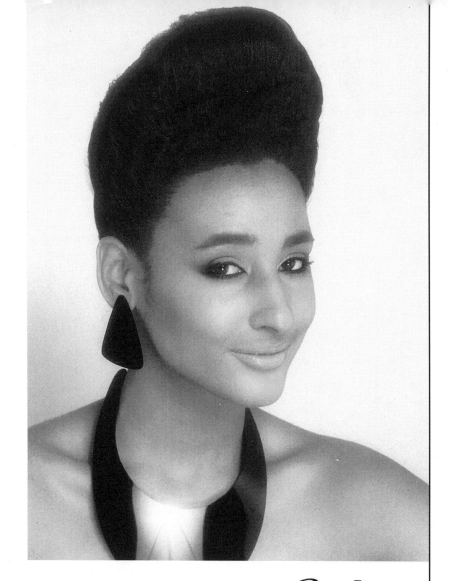

Your HAIR

20

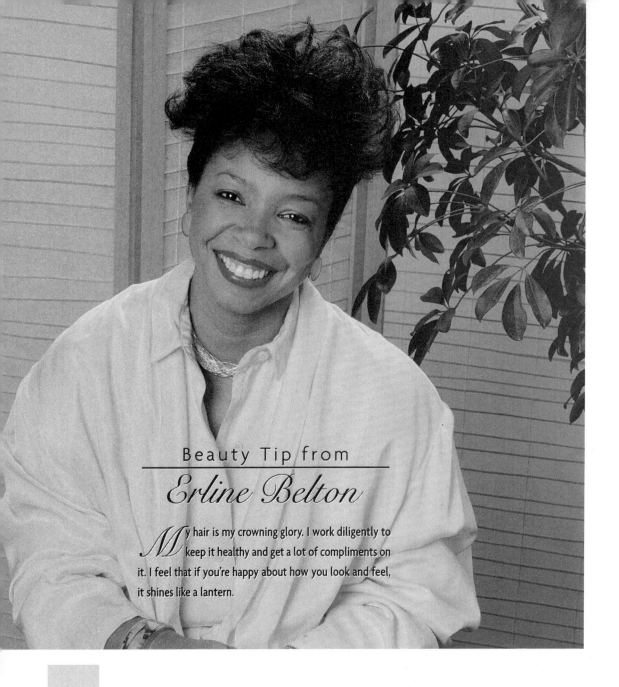

Beauty Tip from

Erline Belton

y hair is my crowning glory. I work diligently to keep it healthy and get a lot of compliments on it. I feel that if you're happy about how you look and feel, it shines like a lantern.

Erline Belton is the president of the Lyceum Group, a consulting firm whose major focus is to influence societal and workplace rethinking, and founder and director of "Living on Purpose," a self-discovery seminar that helps people define their legacy.

While a student at the nation's largest beauty education system, the Wilfred Beauty Academy in New York, I had the opportunity to learn and practice my skills on every type of hair in the world. My first position as a hair stylist was in Macy's department store in New York City. The majority of women whose hair I styled were white, from all parts of the world and with all types of hair textures. This was a learning opportunity, but I wanted experience with black hair.

A friend, Delores, and I decided that the only way we were going to get hands-on experience with African American hair was to work in an African American environment. So I went straight to Harlem. I was hired to work at a prestigious and elegant salon, the Rose Morgan House of Beauty.

Never before, or since, have I seen a beauty salon so elegantly appointed. I learned that the right hairstyle makes a woman feel more confident and secure about her total appearance. Her hair and her makeup communicate attractive and positive images to those around her. Women have told me that when they know they are well made up and their hair is just right, they feel they are on top of the world. They know they feel and look great.

BLACK HAIR IS MANAGEABLE

Don't worry, your hair can readily be managed by you or your hairstylist. Black women's hairstyles and hair management have come full circle. This $4-billion black beauty industry has researched and developed all types of formulas for styling and maintaining black hair.

My past work at the Rose Morgan House of Beauty and the years of experience that have followed have taught me about the various textures and colors, cuts, styles, and maintenance of black hair, which has some great natural features.

NATURAL FEATURES OF BLACK HAIR

1. Black women retain their hair longer as they mature than any other group of people.

2. A black woman can style her hair in more ways—including braids, plaits, and cornrows—than any other woman.

3. Black hair has natural, built-in body owing to its curly wave pattern. African American hair comes in some thirty or more textures, based on tribal origin, from Nubian and Mandingo to African Australian.

THE RIGHT HAIRSTYLE

Today's salon hairstylists are a refreshing new breed of creative, skillful, talented people who can make appropriate suggestions concerning your hair care, as well as cut, curl, and style your hair—all based on your facial shape.

If you consider working with your hair, keep your face in mind. Too much hair moving forward toward the center of your head, with bangs falling into your eyes, will show age on your face more than any other hairstyle. On the other hand, hair moving away from the center of your forehead takes years off your face.

For some reason, many black women wear hairstyles that move their hair forward toward the center of the forehead, making their face appear much older and more mature than it is. Instead, reverse this apparent movement. For example, if you have a low forehead and a short neck, you can give the illusion of adding more height by styling your hair high, with medium curls on your head, and by keeping your hair away from your neck, styling it close to the sides of your head.

On the other hand, when a woman's hair is long, all anyone sees is her head and shoulders; they don't see her neck. If your neck is long and you have a high forehead, style your hair to fall into soft curls, some to the side and some across the forehead in a sculptured fashion.

To help you with styling problems, I have put together a collection of hairstyles that address problems with the neck, forehead, nose, jaw, and chin. As you will see, these styles vary from straight or curly to cornrows and Afros. They are meant to excite your imagination while providing the necessary clues you can employ to camouflage a problem.

In these styles you will not find the exaggerated, short, and wavy marcelled look, the fashionable ornaments and ribbons or gold jewelry adornments, or the pancake and flattop styles. Such styles are neither for you nor for the life you lead. In all cases, remember that *symmetry* and *balance* are the operative words.

HAIR SHAPING

The right haircut and shape are the keys to an ideal hairstyle. African American women must go regularly to a professional beauty salon for shaping and cutting. Some women prefer a barbershop, but I recommend a women's salon. The lines and symmetry for women's hairstyles are entirely different from men's. In cutting and shaping your hair, a professional should take your features and facial shape into consideration. Extreme hairstyles are to be avoided.

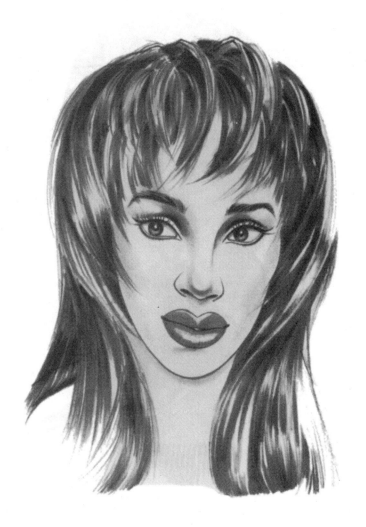

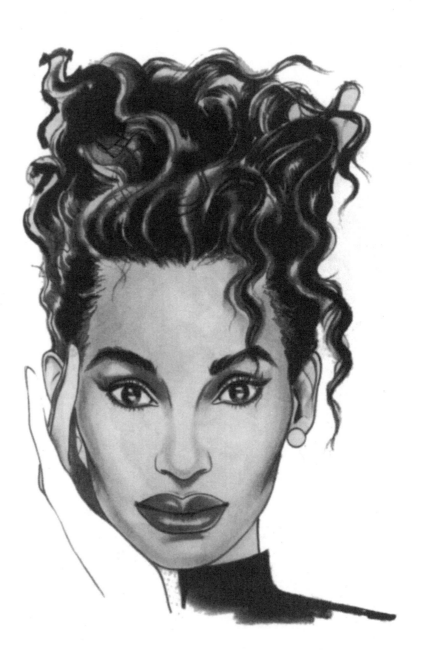

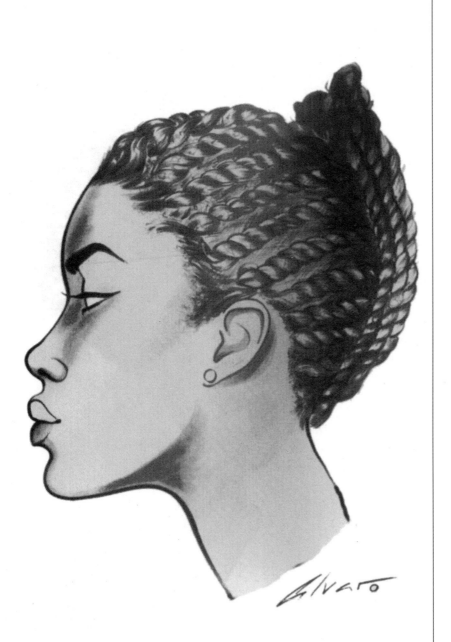

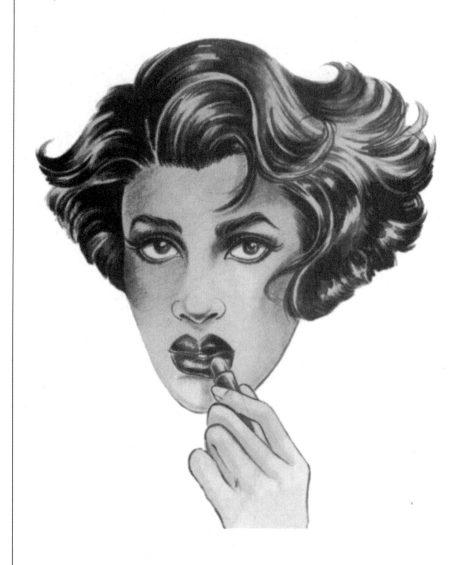

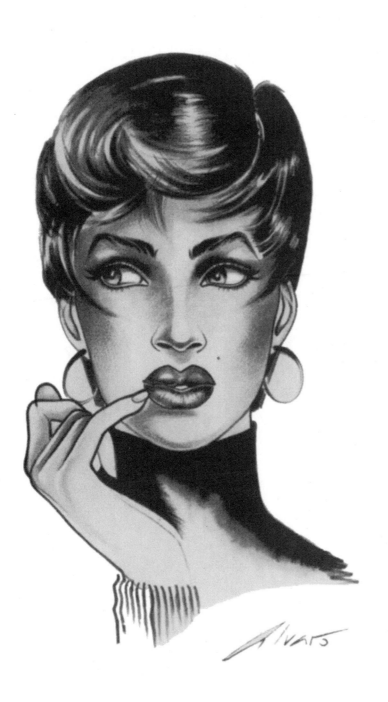

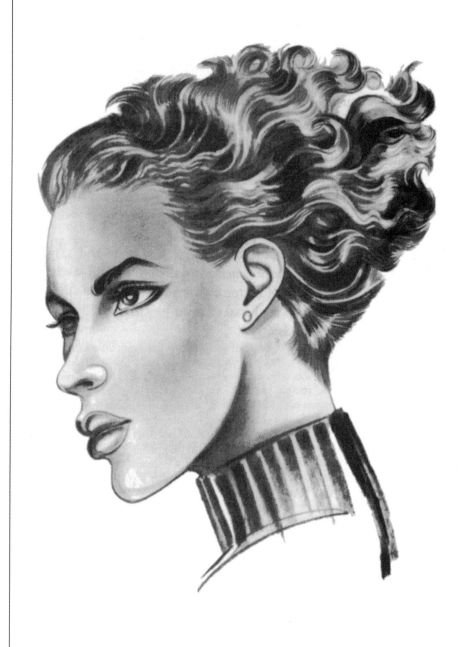

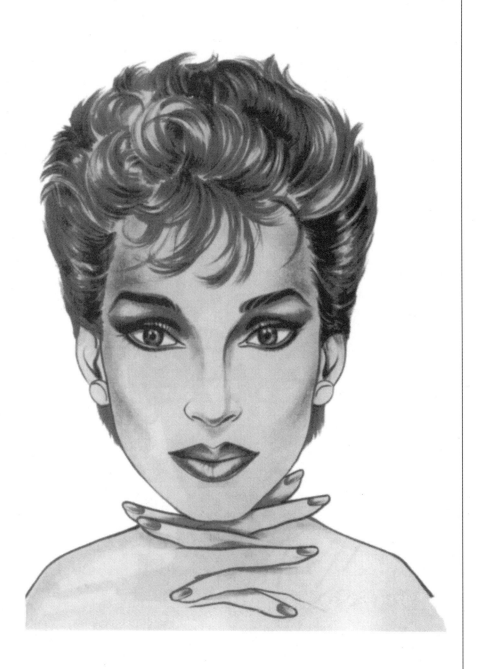

Hair Color

When I was beauty editor at *Ebony* magazine, the editors of *Chain and Drug Store* magazine, a trade publication, asked me, "What were the newest trends in hair grooming products for the black woman of the '90s?" The answer was obvious: the African American woman wanted more color in her life. Women of color wanted to enhance and highlight their otherwise very dark hair. Well, what was perceived as a trend then is now an avalanche. I could not be happier. Today's black woman of the new millennium is throwing off the shackles of dowdy conservatism.

No longer are just black companies preparing hair products for African Americans. The rich bronzes and browns with apricot-cinnamon and chestnut highlights are fabulous, and some blondes do have more fun too. Variety is definitely here!

Natural black hair color comes in some thirty or more gradations, from the ash blonde of Samoa to the flaxen blonde of New Orleans. Like your skin undertone, your hair has a tone that ranges from yellow-gold or yellow-red to red, dark red, or red-brown, and to brown-black. Your skin tone, eye color, and natural hair color are your best guides in choosing a correct hair color. Remember: you have my color chart to help you. You also have help available from your beauty salon hair colorist and the manufacturer's information in the insert and on the back of the hair coloring package.

The best guide to choosing a hair color, however, is a hair strand test, which you can do yourself. Test a strand or section of hair to see how the new color will relate to your eyes and skin. Also determine how the change makes you feel—before going all the way. Take a strand from underneath your outer layer of hair so it won't show if you decide not to proceed. The strand test can be done under the supervision of your hair colorist or at home with an over-the-counter product.

Whichever coloring process you choose—home or salon—there are three basic types of hair color:

Temporary color. These are shampoo-in formulas that are nonalkaline and work gently with the natural chemistry of your hair. Temporary colors are noncoating and will not penetrate the hair shaft. Temporary colors wash out and usually do not contain ammonia, peroxide, or other harmful ingredients.

Semipermanent color. These are designed to harden and coat the outer cuticle shaft of the hair. Semipermanent colors start to rinse off after four to six washings. Some semipermanent color products contain peroxide.

Permanent color. These change the character pigment balance and natural hair color. Permanent hair coloring is best applied in a salon by a professional hair colorist, particularly if you are insecure about your first color change. Permanent hair color products last longer than any other hair change process. Special care for treated hair is advised.

Color crayons. There are some excellent touch-up tools, made of tea, stearate, paraffin, and beeswax. Hair coloring crayons are designed to conceal the roots of your natural hair growth between temporary, semipermanent, and permanent hair colorings. You moisten the crayon and apply it to the hair shaft.

There are other natural and synthetic ways to change your hair color, including special formulas to cover gray hair, color tints, color sprays, mousses, natural henna, and comb-in hair coloring.

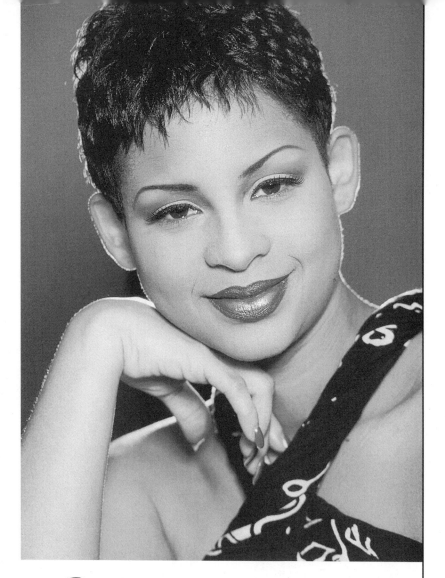

$\mathcal{Y}$OUR **HANDS** ARE LOVELY

21

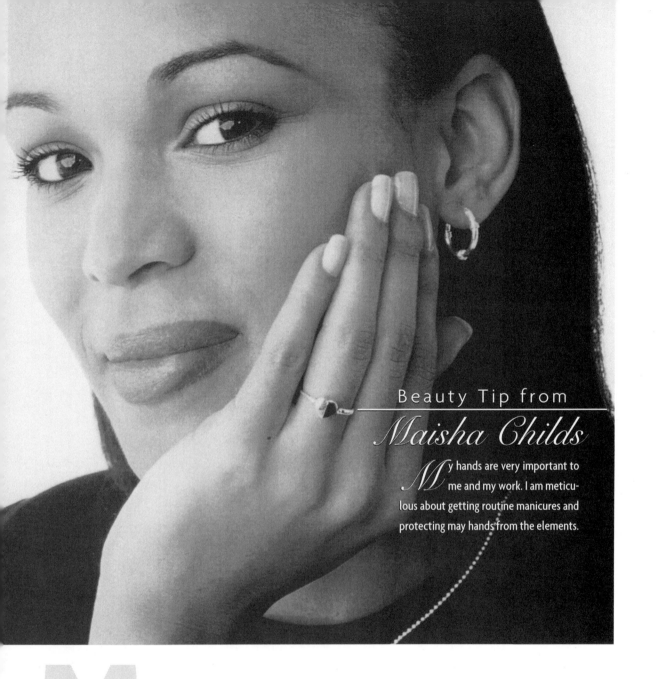

Maisha Childs

*M*y hands are very important to me and my work. I am meticulous about getting routine manicures and protecting may hands from the elements.

Maisha Childs is the wife of Chris Childs, point guard for the New York Knicks. She has many credits that cover a spectrum of diverse roles, as an actress, model, and television personality.

Lovely hands can be the ultimate statement in your total grooming regimen. But making that statement requires proper care.

Your hands are constantly exposed to stresses: weather, pollutants, detergents and other irritating chemicals, and dirt. They get cut, bruised, and scraped. When you clean your hands, you usually wash them in soap and water, removing the limited moisture and oils the body has provided to protect them. Your hands do not have as many oil-producing glands or as much fatty tissue per square inch as does your face. There are no oil glands on the palms of your hands (sweat glands, yes). Thus, washing with drying soaps is more stressful for your hands than you probably realize.

The results of poor hand care can often be seen in the ashen-colored skin between the thumb and index finger, and on the knuckles and cuticles of black women. Regardless of your skin tone, dry-looking skin is unattractive. It shows up more on dark skin, and therefore black skin requires a more intensive hand-care regimen. As you would suppose, the seasons of the year affect your hands differently, and the worst season is winter.

Winter hand care usually means applying an extra-dry hand-cream formula. I do not recommend petroleum jelly, since it gives the hands a greasy, tacky look and feel. It also attracts dirt particles to the hands and under the nails. There are excellent over-the-counter hand-care products to use, but you must use them faithfully.

Proper care of the hands also requires periodic, regular pampering, which includes a regular manicure. Learn from your manicurist about how to care for your hands personally between visits.

YOUR NAILS

Let's look at some important terms before discussing nail health and care. The nail mantle is a protective plate located at the end of the finger. It is made up of the following:

PARTS OF THE NAIL

1. The nail bed, upon which the nail surface rests.
2. The cuticle, a thin outer layer of the nail skin epidermis.

3. The matrix, or formative intercellular tissue of the nail; blood cells nourish the matrix.

4. The lunule, or whitish half-moon shape at the base of the fingernail.

The important, often-abused cuticles serve to protect the nail and keep environmental impurities and germs away from the healthy growing nail.

NAIL-CARE PRODUCTS AND PROCESSES

There are several terms that a manicurist uses in caring for your nails.

TERMS USED IN NAIL CARE

- *Nail bleach.* A salon manicuring cosmetic used to remove stains from under the edges of the fingernail tips.
- *Nail white.* A nail cosmetic used to whiten the free edge of the nail.
- *Nail white pencil.* A pencil containing a hard white chalk, used to whiten the free edge underneath the fingernail tips.
- *Nail enamel or polish.* A fingernail polish in the form of a liquid that forms a colored or transparent coating on fingernails.
- *Nail lacquer.* A thick liquid that forms a high glossy film on your nails.
- *Nail transplants.* Process by which a manicurist cements a broken fingernail to a natural nail.
- *Nail extensions.* Process by which a manicurist applies a premixed material at the juncture of the natural fingernail tip and the silver-foil nail form, forming and sculpting an artificially extended nail.
- *Nail wrappings.* Process by which the manicurist covers the nail's outer tissue, sealing it with a protective nail enamel or glaze, for a smoother, harder, and more durable nail that is then prepared to receive enamel.

You should use special precautions if you are considering artificial nails. Many health-care providers experienced with hand and nail care will agree that artificial nails cause all kinds of problems for nails. Fungus infections and bacterial growth are major concerns.

NAIL HEALTH

A healthy nail grows $1/32$ of an inch each week. Nails grow rapidly until you are thirty, and then as you mature their growth rate decreases to one half the youthful rate. Of course, a good diet, regular exercise, and adequate water consumption will enhance the health of your nails.

Slower-than-normal nail growth can result in excessive thickening of the nails. Breaking, splitting, and peeling can be hereditary or can result from a dietary deficiency or a nutritional imbalance. If any of these conditions worsen, consult your physician or dermatologist before your next manicure.

As strange as it may seem—except to women who have had firsthand experience—physicians with limited, if any, prior experience with black patients sometimes see a dark-skinned woman with heavily pigmented nails (and dark-pigmented gums or lined pigmented eyes) or naturally dark cuticles and conclude that she has an illness—or worse. I am so annoyed with such lazy doctors; I have to assume that they don't care to know more, for the medical data are available, telling them and the world that these are distinct racial features of many healthy African Americans.

Your eyes, mouth, hands, and nails are mirrors of your health, and knowledgeable doctors are able to discern health versus disease. Many normal conditions in blacks are abnormal in whites. Your physician or dermatologist should know this. Make sure the professionals who treat you are skilled, experienced, and knowledgeable about black skin and its conditions.

Also, if at any time you notice that your hands show a reddish yellowing, with a reddish-purple aura against a white background, immediately consult your doctor.

Likewise, if you have infected, sensitive, crusty dark cuticles, swollen and sensitive skin at the sides of the nails and fingertips, skin discolorations, or rashes and fine bumps, you should be concerned and seek medical advice.

HOME CARE OF YOUR NAILS

The use of chemicals—whether taken internally or as topical medications—drastic diet changes, and nail color, polish removers, artificial nails, and nail base coats can often cause nail discoloration, nail breakage, dryness, and general poor nail health. If possible, wear gloves when working in the garden, washing dishes, and so on. Buff your nails on occasion, giving them a relief from the nail base and polish. Be careful with your eating habits and don't go on crash diets. Watch your medication; don't be pill happy, as so many of us are. Good nutrition and proper vitamin supplements will help keep your nails healthy while doing wonders for your entire system.

Regularly consult a professional manicurist. Ask your manicurist to teach you how to care for your hands and nails in between visits. In addition, to help you care for your nails, I have prepared the following basic at-home program.

HAND AND NAIL WARDROBE

You will need a bowl of warm, sudsy water; a bowl of clear water; and towels. Then gather the following items and use them in the order indicated.

1. *Polish remover.* A fragrance-free, oil-based formula without acetone.
2. *Cotton balls.* Large balls for nail cleaning and polish removal.
3. *Nail file.* Wood or metal for shaping and cleaning.
4. *Cream or liquid cuticle remover.* Aids in the removal of dead skin around cuticles.
5. *Cuticle stick.* To gently push back the cuticles.
6. *Base coat.* Holds the color on the nail.
7. *Nail polish.* Coloring as follows: cream and frost for all occasions; high lacquer gloss for glamorous occasions.
8. *Top coat.* Seals the color in and protects the surface.

You should also have a hand cream designed for manicure use and cuticle cream for nightly cuticle protection.

Your nail color should match your lipstick—that is, blue nails do not go with red lipstick. Pick up your fashion cues from your garments. Also, consult my color chart.

QUICK TOUCH-UP PROCEDURES

There are two possible methods. The first is to remove any old polish and apply nail cream, then buff your nails. The second method is to remove the polish, apply a clear base coat, and a tinted polish, then add a top coat.

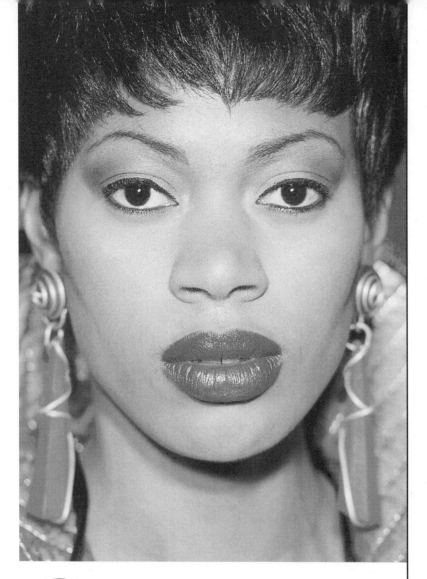

QUICK TIPS FOR THE **LOOK** YOU WANT

NaN22

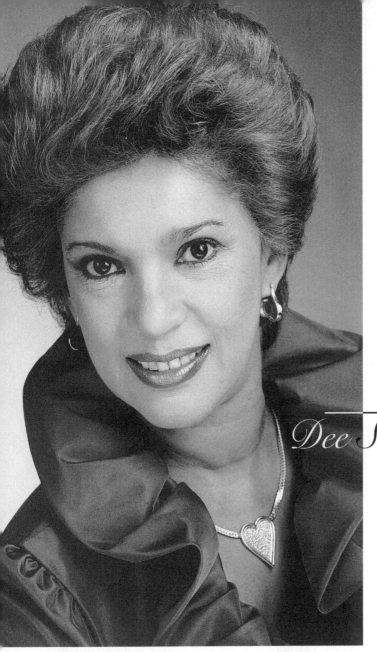

Beauty Tip from
Dee Simmons-Edelstein

I'm always on the go and sometimes change my plans on a moment's notice. I always have to be an example for the models that I represent, so I have created various grooming techniques ranging from quick touch-ups to the full gamut of glamour.

Dee Simmons-Edelstein is vice president of Ophelia DeVore Associates and the executive director of Grace Del Marco. In her role as director, she has been responsible for launching the careers of some of today's top black models. Dee is also the producer and host of her TV cable show *The Dee Simmons Show*.

The majority of black women do not wear color makeup, or wear only very little. Probably as many as 65 percent do not wear those wonderful and exciting eye colors and blushes.

That means that lipstick and foundation are probably the only colors you usually wear. So this is where you begin and on what you build. In fact, too much makeup is unattractive. Too much unblended makeup seen in daylight is overstated. Keep the sparkle and pizzazz for special evening affairs. But now that you know how to add color skillfully and beautifully, it's time to enjoy and enhance your natural beauty.

Think of all the role models for both your beliefs and your lifestyle. For instance, there are such beauties as the TV stars Phylicia Rashad and Sheryl Lee Ralph, who are never overly made up. There is a naturalness to their fully made-up faces, and their eyes never have excessive color, yet they look lovely.

There are many appropriate models for the look of successful African American women. For example, look at Dr. Mae Jamison, the first black female astronaut, and take a look at the wives of the black mayors of major cities; observe the wives of our black fire and police commissioners. See the wives of football or basketball stars. Look at professional women athletes too. The women who are presidents of black colleges or presidents of major black organizations—they all make excellent role models. They are never overly made up.

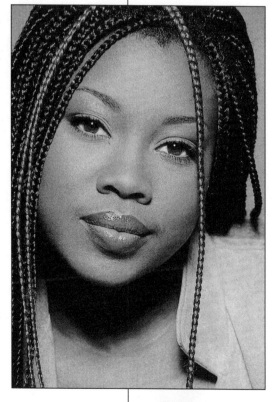

*L*ESS IS BETTER

Refined, secure black women show themselves by making a clear, natural, never overcolored statement to the world. You are about serious business. You are striving to be the best you can—at work, in your social affairs, at home, and in church. Others should notice you because of the quality of your performance, not through garish makeup or inappropriate use of color.

Now, let's review various makeup applications and techniques so that you can determine which one fits your lifestyle best.

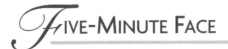

Five-Minute Face

FOLLOW THESE STEPS

1. Cleanse.
2. Tone.
3. Moisturize.
4. Add foundation.
5. Set foundation.
6. Do eyes: one color on eyelids.
7. Apply mascara.
8. Brush eyebrows.
9. Add lipstick color.

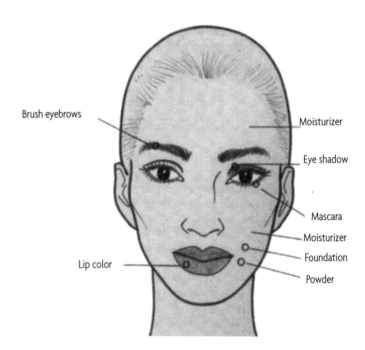

$\mathscr{T}$EN-MINUTE FACE

FOLLOW THESE STEPS

1. Cleanse.

2. Tone.

3. Moisturize.

4. Add foundation.

5. Apply powder to set foundation.

6. Do eyes: apply eye concealer, highlight brow bone with color; apply fashion eye color to area closest to eyelash; apply eyeliner, mascara; brush eyebrows and apply brow pencil.

7. Apply blusher.

8. Apply lip color.

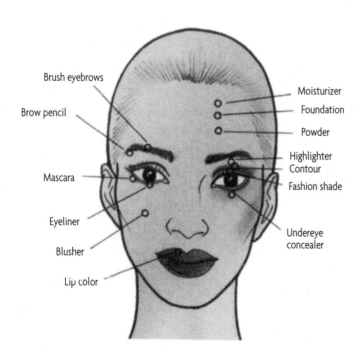

Fifteen-Minute Face

FOLLOW THESE STEPS

1. Cleanse.
2. Tone.
3. Moisturize.
4. Apply undereye concealer.
5. Apply foundation.
6. Apply powder to set foundation.
7. Do eyes: for rainbow eyes, apply fashion shade to under corner of eye, highlight the center point of eyelid, apply eyeliner to top and bottom lids; use brow brush, brow pencil, mascara.
8. Do cheeks: contour the cheek area underneath the cheekbone and then apply blusher on top of cheekbone, blending down to contour.
9. Do lips: use lip pencil to line lips, add lip color with lip brush, and add a touch of lip gloss.

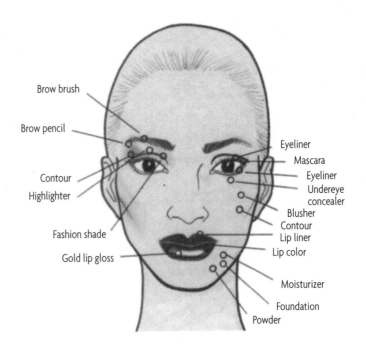

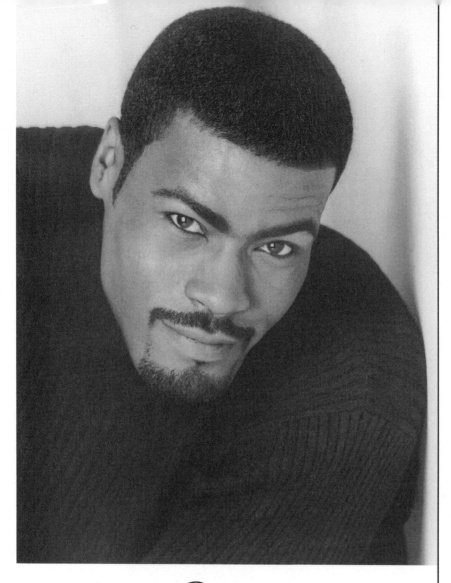

∫KINCARE AND GROOMING FOR **MEN**

23

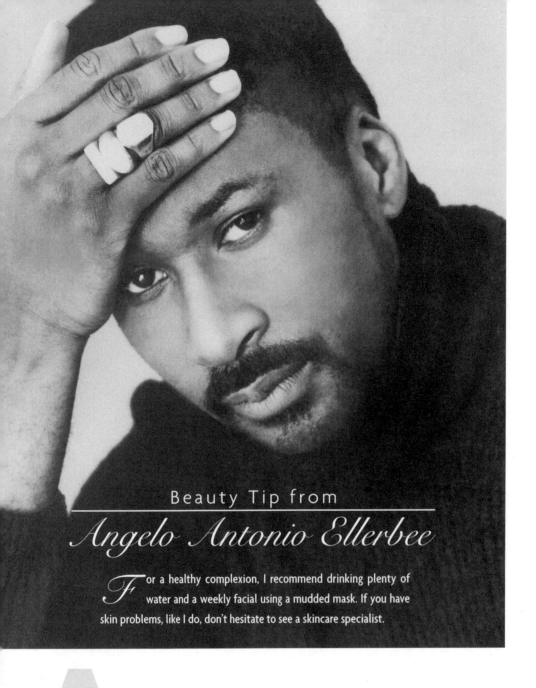

Beauty Tip from

Angelo Antonio Ellerbee

For a healthy complexion, I recommend drinking plenty of water and a weekly facial using a mudded mask. If you have skin problems, like I do, don't hesitate to see a skincare specialist.

Angelo Antonio Ellerbee is president and founder of Double Xposure and Angelo Ellerbee Group, which encompass public relations, artist development, and artist management. He is responsible for creating superstar images for some of the industry's most notable celebrities and is the author of *What's Your Excuse?*

It is women who more often than not choose the clothes that men wear, and men more often "dress up" to please women than other men. Women are also more inclined to buy and read a book like this. Consequently, I include this chapter on men with the hope that you will share it with the men in your life.

More and more, though, men are realizing that proper grooming is not a luxury or simply a personal desire. It is a necessity. Men of color are finding themselves in professional careers where appearance is a critical element of success. They find themselves in positions that call for a suit and tie, such as business meetings, and to be photographed for print media and for television, as well as for social occasions. Whatever the reason, this is a basic skincare and grooming guide for men who want to look their best and for those who want the most sensible solutions for dealing with their particular needs and problems.

RAZOR BUMPS AND OTHER SKIN PROBLEMS

Razor bumps happen when very curly and wiry facial hair, cut at the wrong angle, curves over and into the skin. These bumps are itchy, painful, and can become infected. Once they become infected they can result in keloids— scar tissue—and leave marks and pits in the skin. These razor bumps pose chronic problems for many men and lead many of them to decide to grow beards, opting not to shave at all. Beards can look great, but you should wear one because you want to and not because you feel you have to. Alternatively, there are some shaving techniques whereby you can have a clean-shaven look without the discomfort of razor bumps.

There are preconditioners—gels, foams, liquids, and steam—that soften the beard and set it up for cutting. There are razors with special heads and blades that cut hairs at such an angle that they are less likely to curl over and into the skin. If you have a difficult beard and are susceptible to razor bumps, a single- or twin-blade razor, or a straight-edge razor in the hands of your barber, is best. Many black men, though, find that electric razors nick, cause bumps, and irritate sensitive skin. Curly hair should be shaved in one direction. The electric razor does not cut hair in one direction, and this is why it causes problems. Some men try depilatories in their attempt to avoid shaving problems. If this is your choice, use those designed for sensitive black skin and capable of removing hair without irritation and burning. Some of the products good for preconditioning your skin for shaving are razor burn products, with antibiotic cream and mild hydrocortisone.

BEARDS

If you are going to wear a beard, it should be regularly cleaned, conditioned, brushed or combed, and designed for your facial bone structure. Actually, a beard helps keep the skin looking younger because the hairs protect the skin from sun damage. The hairs will also keep the skin from folding, therefore the skin will have fewer wrinkles. Acne problems are also less of a problem for men with beards. Consult a good barber to determine the appropriate shape of the beard for your bone structure.

A SKINCARE REGIMEN

Attending to your face requires but minutes a day. Refer to chapters 1 through 3 to learn how to establish a skincare regimen that suits your skin type. Cleanse, tone, and moisturize are the key steps to healthy and great-looking skin for men too.

I strongly recommend that men treat themselves to facials periodically. Not only are they good for keeping the skin moisturized and healthy, but they also help relieve tension. Getting a facial can offer you a peaceful time when you can relax those facial muscles. Adequate sleep, plenty of water, annual medical checkups, and sound daily nutritional habits are important as well.

HAIR GROOMING

There has never been a time when the African American male has had more hairstyle options. Yet this very fact has added an issue every professional adult male must address if he wishes to move effectively and smoothly from the boardroom or TV station into the playing field or other social setting.

Just as the style and color of your clothes can admit you to or keep you out of certain places, so can your hairstyle. Certain hairstyles are acceptable in the entertainment world but not in the executive boardrooms of Wall Street and Park Avenue. Styles that make you "hip" in social situations may be counterproductive in terms of your business career. The style that is in fashion may also be inappropriate for your face.

When it comes to choosing a hairstyle, look for one that will fit the most critical aspects of your life. For example, if you choose the latest fad styles, you are making a clear nonconservative, nonbusiness statement, and you should expect to be viewed, if not treated, accordingly.

The best general hairstyle is still the classic look, a reasonably cropped style, which tapers gently downward to the sides and nape of the neck, with a clean neckline. This style can be just as natural and appropriate by wearing your hair somewhat fuller overall or by employing gentle, full waves with the hair somewhat longer at the nape of the neck. Another variation is to have the temples fuller and nape fuller. This style is great if you have large ears or if they stand away from the head. Having a fuller top elongates the face.

If you are patterned bald or balding, wear your hair closely cropped. This reduces the look of baldness. To retard the balding process, cleanse your hair at least once a week with a shampoo formulated for your type of hair. Massage your hair daily with your fingertips to stimulate the blood flow. This will help feed the hair follicles.

When shampooing your hair, always apply a conditioner after shampooing and wash it out after about five minutes. Leaving it in longer will not hurt, but it will not do any more good. Before your hair is styled, it should always be shampooed. If you have coarse hair, you may want a mild relaxer applied before your shampoo and styling. But if you use a relaxer, be sure to use an acid-neutralized shampoo.

Do not forget that hair texture for black males comes in as many varieties as black skin color, and it will therefore need different treatments. If you want a modern rather than a classic look, have your hair processed with a curly perm, giving it a sheen and high manageability. If you use chemicals on your hair, it becomes more susceptible to damage; therefore, such hair must be properly conditioned and periodically rested from chemicals to maintain its health.

But whatever your hair type or perceived problem, there is a product to assist you, from relaxers to curlers, from toupees to weaves, from transplants to glue-ons or braids—all giving you the look of a natural, full head of hair. Think first about the look you want and its affect on both your total image and your lifestyle before choosing it.

Conclusion

I have found that everyone seems to have something to say about the African American woman, but no one seems to be listening to her. Cosmetics companies and general market beauty and fashion magazines tend to take too narrow a view of both black beauty culture and black style, often pursuing their own policies and points of view, rather than acting as true reflections of our complex African American generation. Our generation is different from previous ones. The industry is finally recognizing the African American woman's twenty-first-century beauty needs and realizing that she doesn't have just one beauty image appearance; she has many beauty looks.

African American women have, within their souls, potentialities that can be discovered and nurtured to help them become more attractive, more interesting, and more appealing persons. *The African American Woman's Guide to Successful Makeup and Skincare* was written and designed specifically to help you make the most of these potentialities so that you can achieve success and happiness, both in your work and in your personal life.

I have had the opportunity to travel all over this world to observe beautiful women of African heritage. I've enjoyed sharing with you my experiences, and you have taught me to respect and appreciate your ageless beauty.

This basic beauty guide expresses the needs and wants of the twenty-first-century African American woman, who is dynamic and assured, with strong family values, by providing perspectives on her beauty and her total beauty image in the workplace and at home.

You are the intended audience of *The African American Woman's Guide to Successful Makeup and Skincare*—women with buying power and influence, who care for their style of living and that of their families.

I look forward to meeting you soon.

Alfred Fornay

Acknowledgments

To my supportive sisters, Beverly and Elizabeth; nieces, Sharmyn, Julie, Darla, Carla, Sherry; and nephew, Troy.

Mentors:

John H. Johnson
Benjamin Wright
Elsie Archer
Dr. Alfred Sloan
Hurley Phillips
Joseph Merriweather
Rose Morgan
John Ledes
Anthony B. Colletti

Carole Hall, editor in chief, African American Books, John Wiley & Sons, Inc.; Tony Rose, publisher, Amber Books; Yvonne Rose, senior editor, Amber Books; Terrie Williams of the Terrie Williams Agency; Kimberly Monroe, John Wiley & Sons, Inc.; Shelly Perron; John Ledes, Samuel P. Peabody, Joan Bowser, Bob Tate, Edward Lewis, Clarence Smith, Susan L. Taylor, Ionia Dunn-Lee, Marcia Ann Gillespie, Mike J. Bramwell, Byron Barnes, Constance White, Brian Basil Daley, Naomi Sims, Alex, Valerie Bennett, Earle Holman, Ashley Hall, John Blassingame, Eddie and Grace Phipps, Edythe Karr, Sybil Gooden, Fred Dillon, Iman, Emmitt Dudley, Gwendolyn Nicholas, Carolyn Florence, Brian Hayes Copeland, Georginia G. Hill, Terry Ivory, Kelly Rollins, Bernice Coleman, Wanda J. Baskerville, Gloria Pflanz, Darrin Patrick, D'angelo Thompson, Lawrence Burchall, Kelvin Wall, Kendal Aegri, Sherry Bronfman, Audrey Bernard, Barbara Harris, Lu Willard, Evelyn Cunningham, Dr. Gloria E. A. Toote, Bernice Calvin, Milton Scott, Wentworth Christopher, Bert Emanuel, Sheila Evers, Regina Fleming, Aunt Lois, Walter Greene, Therez Fleetwood, Ronald Lihurd, Alan Price, Roy Hastick, Ruth Sanchez, Emel Lindsay Cross, Jessica Harris, Mary Garthe, Betty Johnson, Bernice Whistleton, Ernest Lee, Joan Murray, Tony, Michael, James Harris, Smiler Haynes, Rudy Townsel, Kathleen Myer Lane, Winston Isaacs, Jacqueline Champagnie, and Kowan Choi.

Amber Books special acknowledgments:

Tony Rose, publisher and editorial director

Samuel P. Peabody, associate publisher

Terry Ivory, editor

Yvonne Rose, editor

Terrie Williams, Terrie Williams Agency

Lisa Liddy, cover and interior design

Wayne "Zoom" Summerlin, cover, flip cover, and interior models photographer

Alvaro, illustrator

Cover model, Jeneen Willmore

Christopher Michael, cover model makeup artist

Randy Stodghill, cover model hair stylist

Jewel Shannon, cover model fashion stylist

Dwight Carter, before and after and cosmetic tool model photographer

Byron Barnes, before and after and cosmetic tool makeup artist

Wayne Parham, interior and cosmetic tool model photographer

Interior models: Zu-baydah, Cindy

Before and after models: Egypt Lawson, Beverly English, Elizabeth Wilburn, Nilsa Graham

Flip cover models: Cecily Witcher, Judith Riley, Ericka T. Moran, Greer Alexander

Shonnette, flip cover models makeup artist

Yvonne Rose, flip cover photo production coordinator

Therez Fleetwood, flip cover photo design

Ashley Hall, flip cover fashion stylist

Jatawn Avanti, flip cover models fashion stylist/dresser

Roger Gary, flip cover models designer

Jeanne Moutoussamy-Ashe, photographer for Rita Ewing (chapter 4)

Doug Bizzaro, photographer for Eishia Brightwell (chapter 9)

The models—Vanessa Hope, Miata, Linda Bossfield, Cleo, Akia, Angela Louise, Etta, Stacy, Tamika Lovett, Mia, Zubaidah, Patience, Jacqueline, Janime, Deloris, Cathy, Taija, DeeDee, Charlie, Yvette, Carla, Nina, Deann, Shanish, Clara, Shyvonne, Chantal, Amena, Curbeon, Susan, Anjette, Carla, Mary, Pam Moran, Nakia, Barbara Hope, Stacy, Sheba, Damasa, Angela-Louise, Debbie, Raj, Naemah, Andrea Renee, Ericka Tracy, Andrea Rene, Anjette, Kenny, Rochelle, Raymond Patterson, and Paula Johnson

As always, Amber Books gratefully acknowledges those whose time, patience, help, and advice have contributed to the success of our literary efforts: Donna Beasley, founder, the Chicago Black Book Fair and Conference, the IBBMEC; the nation's African American bookstores; our wholesalers and distributors; the black weekly and national media; Yvonne Rose, whose love and friendship for the illustrious Alfred Fornay brought him to Amber Books; and Alfred Fornay who knows black women, and loves black women everywhere.

Index